Dental Caries

Edited by Efka Zabokova Bilbilova

Published in London, United Kingdom

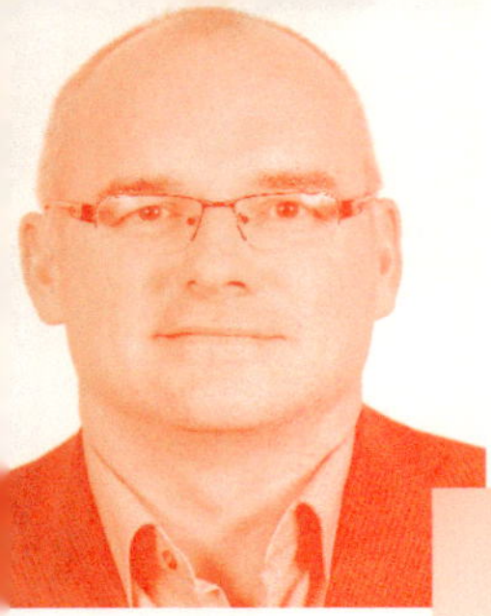
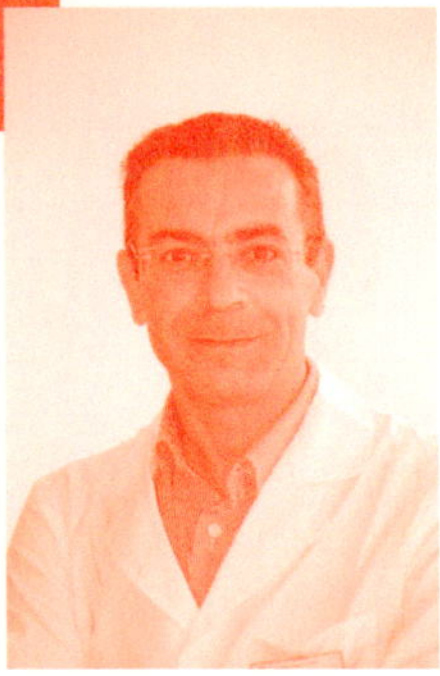
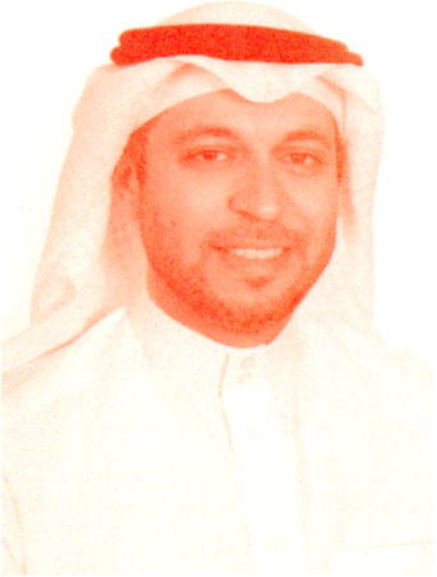
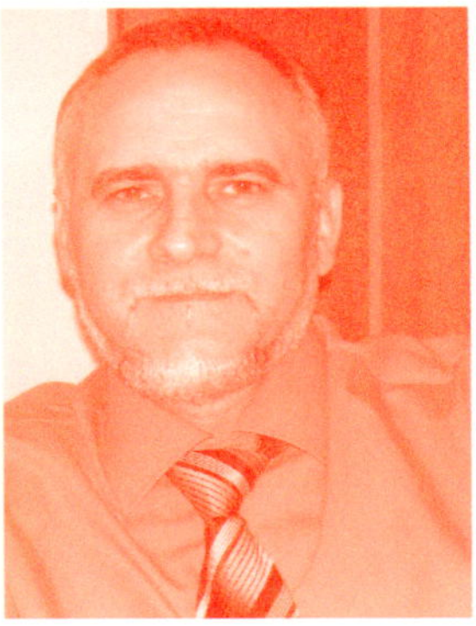
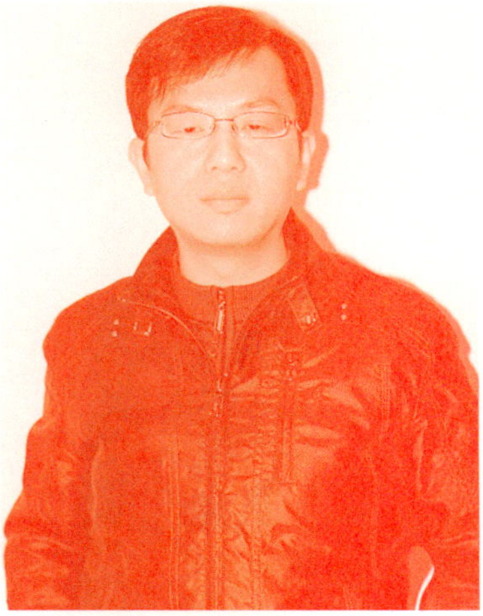
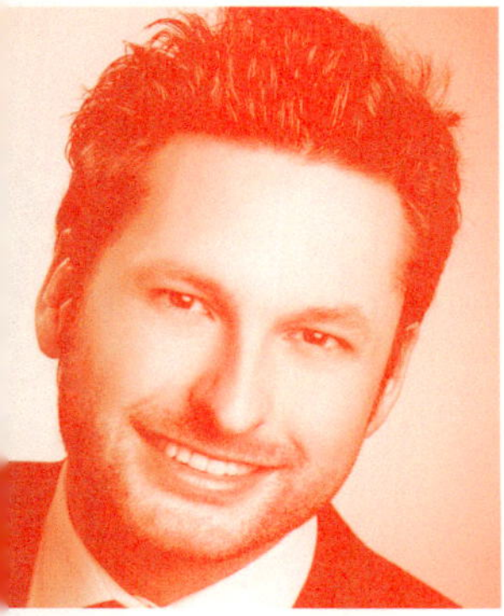
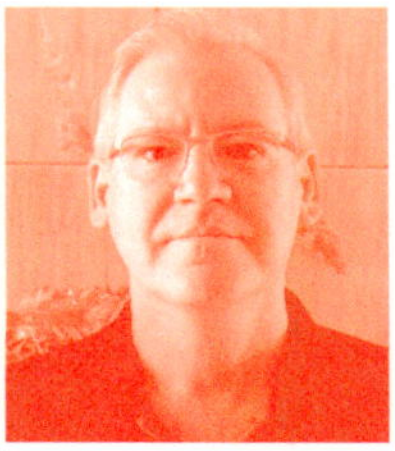

IntechOpen

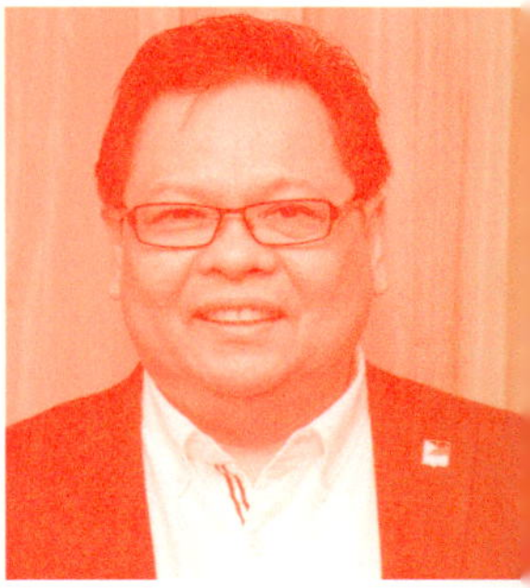
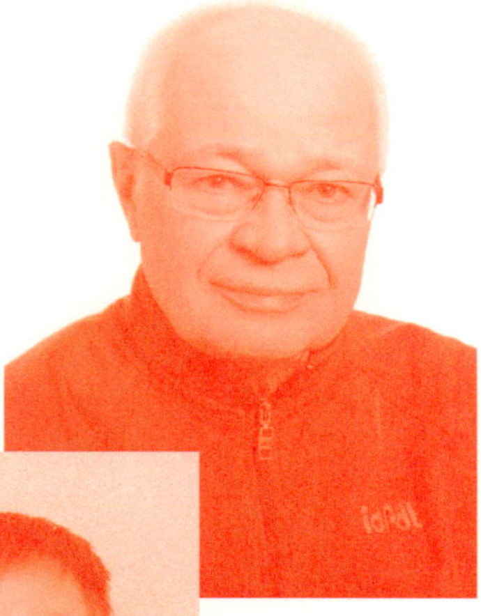
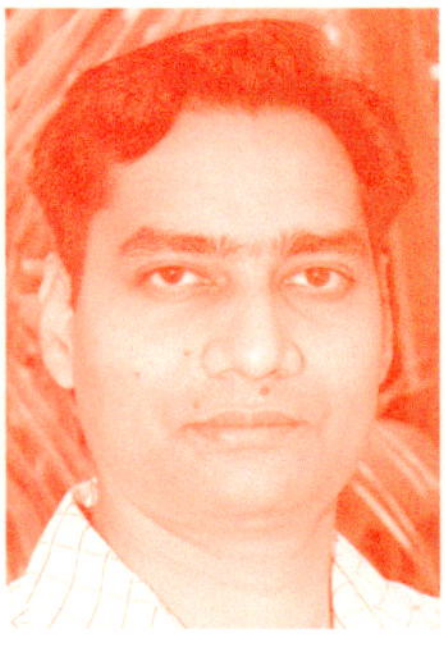
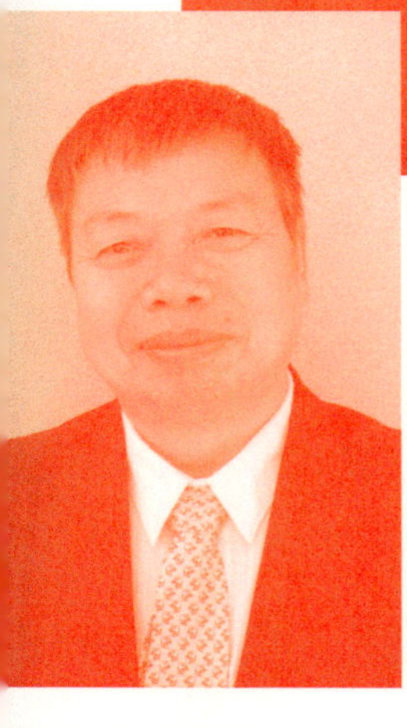
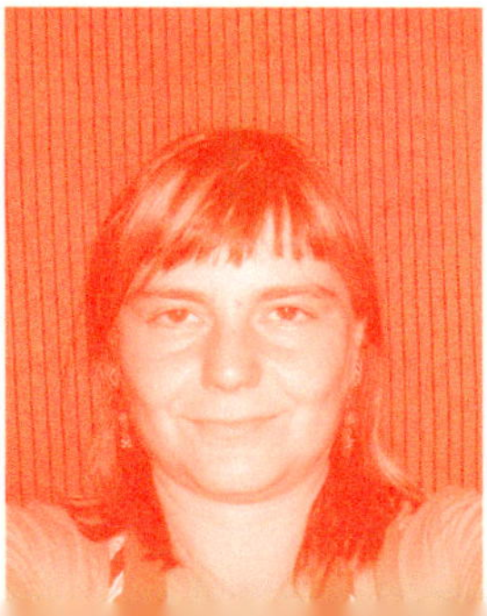
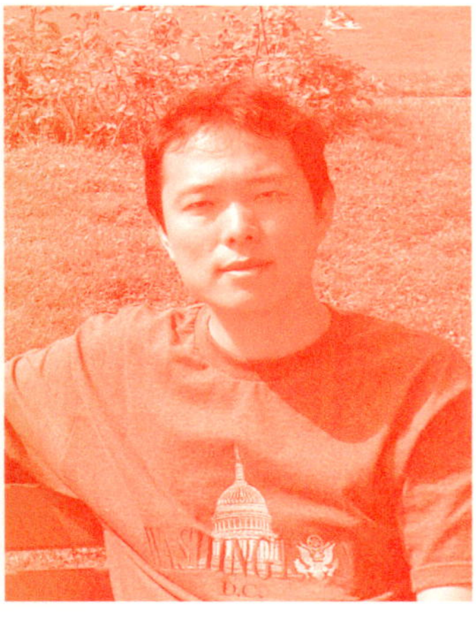

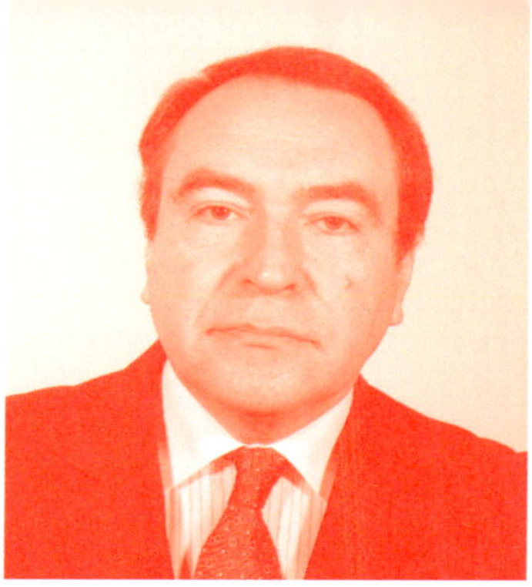
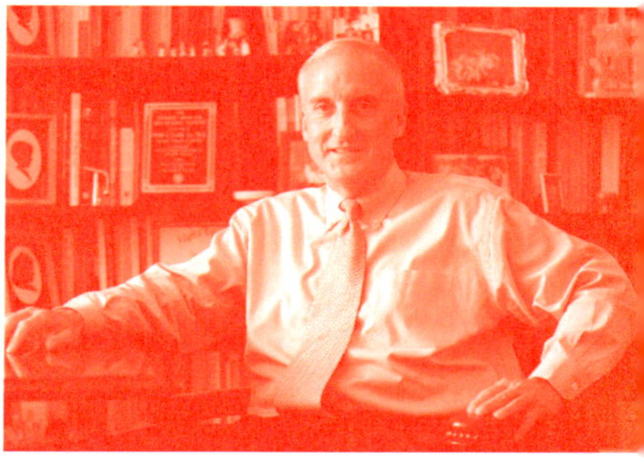
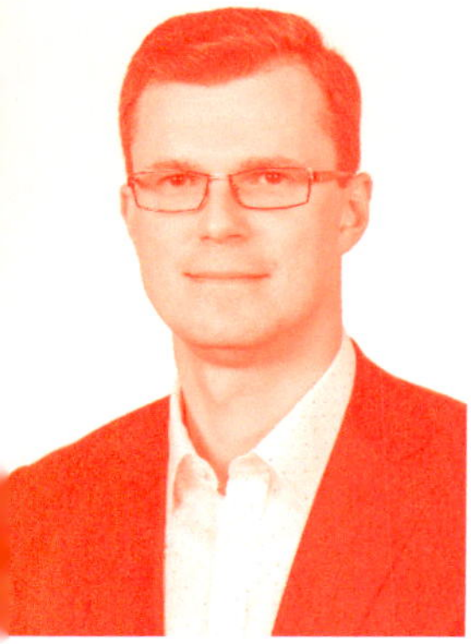
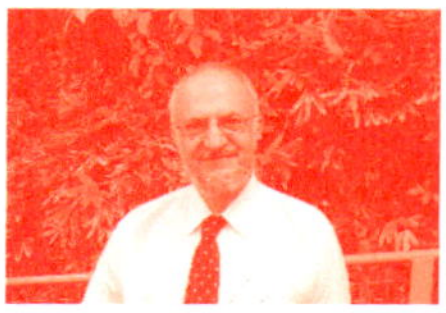
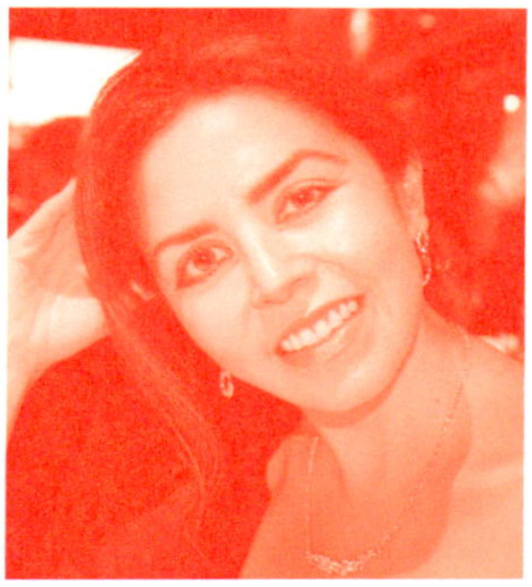

Supporting open minds since 2005

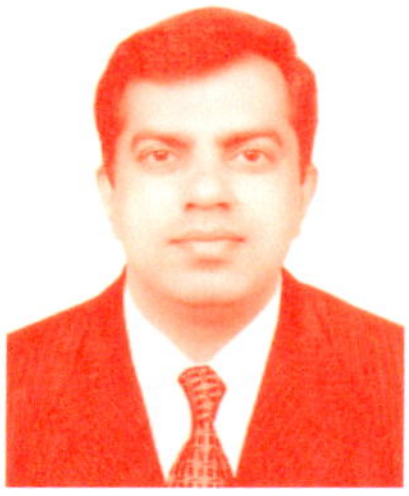
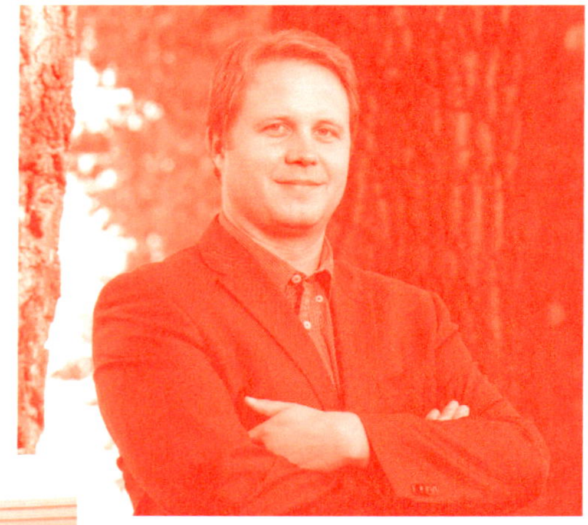
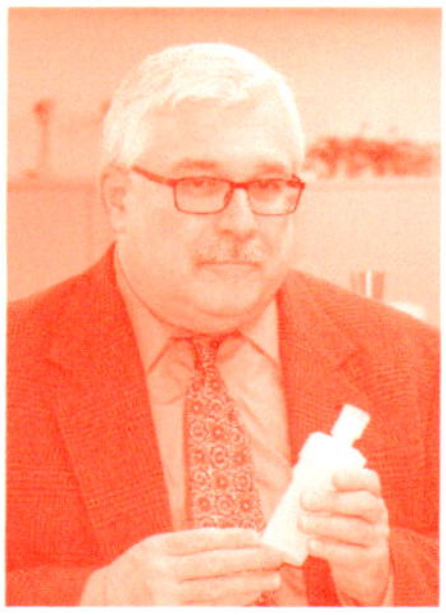
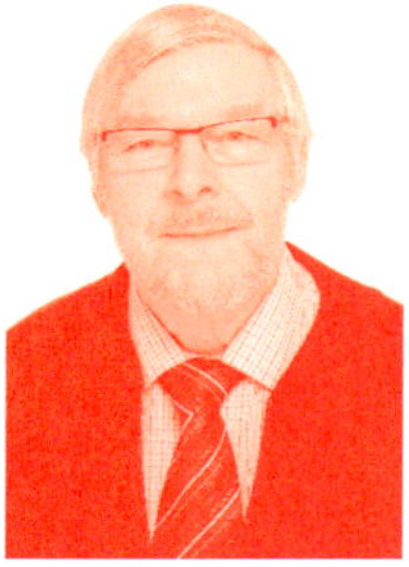
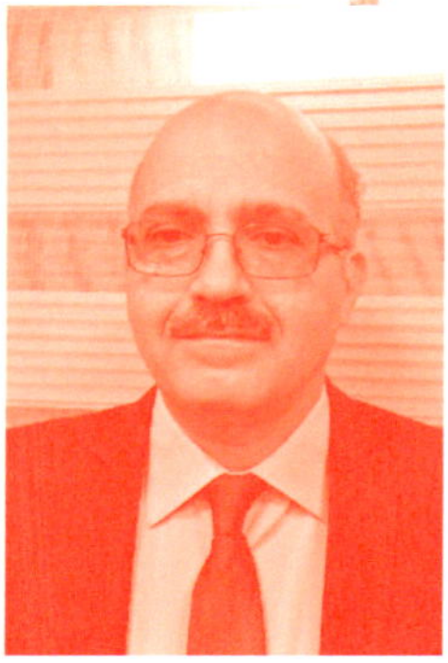
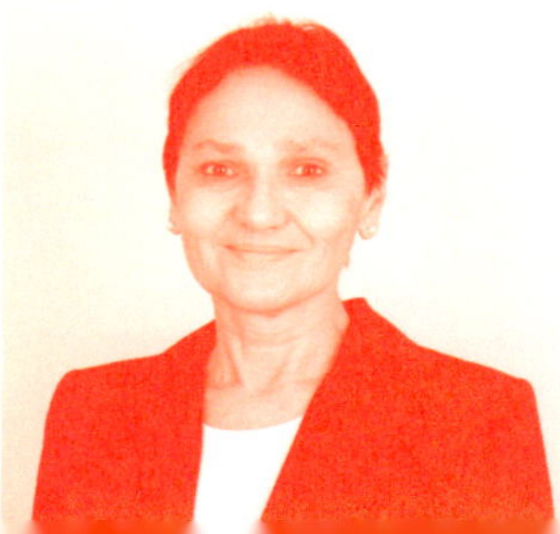
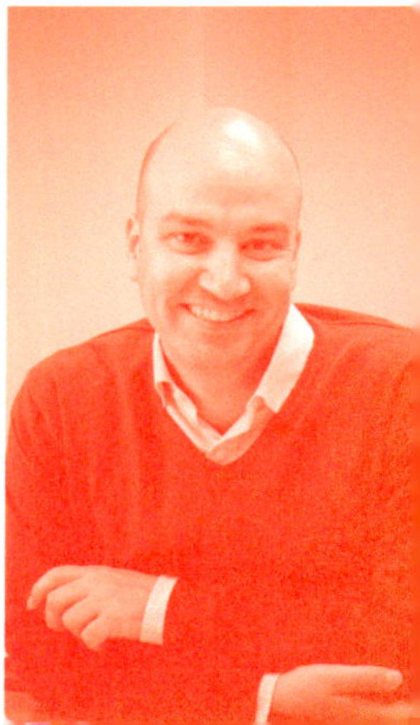

Dental Caries
http://dx.doi.org/10.5772/intechopen.89295
Edited by Efka Zabokova Bilbilova

Contributors
Berna Kuter, Feng Luo, Qianbing Wan, Haiyang Sun, Beena M. S., Ana Claudia Rodrigues Chibinski, Efka Zabokova Bilbilova, Marilen P. Balolong, Emilija Stefanovska, Michael Antonio F. Mendoza

First published in London, United Kingdom, 2021 by IntechOpen
IntechOpen is the global imprint of INTECHOPEN LIMITED, registered in England and Wales, registration number: 11086078, 5 Princes Gate Court, London, SW7 2QJ, United Kingdom
Printed in Croatia

British Library Cataloguing-in-Publication Data
A catalogue record for this book is available from the British Library

Additional hard and PDF copies can be obtained from orders@intechopen.com

Dental Caries
Edited by Efka Zabokova Bilbilova
p. cm.
Print ISBN 978-1-83968-114-1
Online ISBN 978-1-83968-115-8
eBook (PDF) ISBN 978-1-83968-116-5

For EU product safety concerns:
IN TECH d.o.o., Prolaz Marije Krucifikse Kozulić 3, 51000 Rijeka, Croatia, info@intechopen.com or visit our website at intechopen.com.

Meet the editor

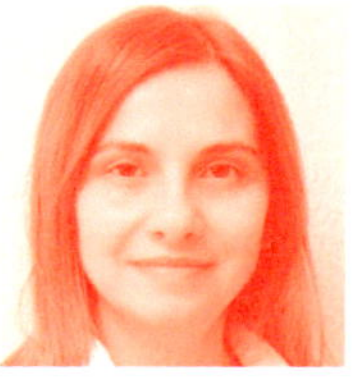

Dr. Efka Zabokova Bilbilova received a BS in Dentistry from the "Ss. Cyril and Methodius" University, Skopje, Republic of Macedonia, in 1997. She obtained an MS in Pediatric and Preventive Dentistry from the same university with a thesis on "The role of salivary urea and bicarbonate on the appearance of dental caries." Dr. Bilbilova received a Ph.D. in 2010, defending the doctoral thesis: "Inhibition on demineralization on enamel around the orthodontic braces during the treatment: in vivo and in vitro study." She specialized in the Department of Pediatric and Preventive Dentistry at the Faculty of Dentistry in 2002. Currently, she is an Associate Professor in the Faculty of Dentistry, Department of Pediatric and Preventive Dentistry, "Ss. Cyril and Methodius" University. She was a visiting researcher at the Institute of Biomedical Research, Medical Faculty, University of Nis, Serbia (2008 and 2010), where she worked on a project to qualitatively evaluate the remineralization potential of different topic material on early enamel lesions. Dr. Bilbilova is also an active member of the Macedonian Dental Association (MDA), Balkan Stomatological Society (BaSS), International Association of Pediatric Dentistry (IAPD), and World Dental Federation (FDI). For her professional work, she received Macedonian Medical Association Acknowledgements in 2001 and the Macedonian Dental Association (2011 and 2014). In 2019 Dr. Bilbilova received acknowledgement of the Faculty of Dentistry at the "Ss. Cyril and Methodius" University in Skopje. She has published more than 210 national and international scientific articles, book chapters, and monographs in the field of pediatric and preventive dentistry as well as buffer systems in saliva and demineralization-remineralization in teeth. She is also an editorial board member for several reputable journals.

Contents

Preface

This book is a compilation of chapters that brings together clinical data on dental caries to provide dental students and practitioners updated information about dental caries, their consequences, and their appropriate treatment.

An understanding of how cavities form is needed to determine treatment procedures and to assess the risk of disease development. Dental caries are of vital concern to all dentists. Their management is central to daily work in dental offices because caries are ubiquitous in all populations, lesion development is lifelong, and caries are the most common cause of tooth loss.

This book begins with Chapter 1, "Introductory Chapter: Dental Biofilms Associated with Caries," in which Dr. Emilija Stefanovska discusses dental biofilm, which is a proven complex biostructure of microorganisms that is the primary etiological factor for the development of the two most common diseases in the oral cavity: caries and periodontal diseases. The biofilm related to dental caries functions in several ways. It is a site of bacterial proliferation and growth, a location of acid/base regulation at the tooth surface, and a reservoir for calcium ion exchange between the tooth and the saliva. The chapter also discusses dental indices, which are a numerical expression for assessing the prevalence and incidence of certain dental conditions as well as determining the need for treatment. Today, dental indices are used to assess both individual and group oral health and disease status. They can be simple, measuring only the presence or absence of a condition, or they can be cumulative, measuring all evidence of a condition, past and present. There are also so-called irreversible indices, which measure conditions that will not change, such as dental caries. Reversible indices, in turn, note changing conditions, such as the amount of dental plaque accumulation.

Chapter 2, "Dietary Factors, Salivary Parameters, and Dental Caries," gives information about dietary factors in the initiation and progression of dental caries. Diet and oral microflora are connected to the formation of caries along with host factors such as salivary composition and flow. Fermentable carbohydrates appear to be the only dietary component capable of causing caries. All fermentable dietary carbohydrates, especially sucrose, are potentially cariogenic, but sucrose is generally accepted as the most cariogenic dietary factor. Sucrose consumption has been associated most consistently with the frequency of dental caries in humans. The author provides clear information on the dental caries process. The initial lesion will continue to lose mineral if treatment is not initiated, and the acidic challenge is unabated. The progressive dissolution of enamel and loss of enamel surface structure eventually give rise to a frank carious lesion and the deterioration of dental health. This chapter also provides information about saliva and its components, which play an important role in maintaining oral and especially dental health. Saliva accomplishes its mechanical cleaning and protective functions through various physical and biochemical mechanisms. Saliva has a buffer capacity that neutralizes acids in the mouth. The carbonic acid/bicarbonate system is the most important buffer in stimulated saliva due to its higher concentration.

In Chapter 3, "Characterization and Virulence of *Candida* Isolated from Children with Dental Caries and Its Susceptibility to Various Antimicrobial Agents," Dr. M.S. Beena examines the association of *Candida* with early colonization of cariogenic microorganisms leading to tooth decay. The author reports on the characterization of *Candida* from dental plaque in children with dental caries and studies virulence factors and antimicrobial activity of coconut oil, probiotics, 0.2% chlorhexidine, and ketoconazole against *C. albicans*. Dr. Beena shows that chlorhexidine and coconut oil have significant antimicrobial activity and scientifically proves the antifungal activity of chlorhexidine, coconut oil, and probiotics. The author also shows that the antifungal activities of coconut oil are greater than those of probiotics against *C. albicans*.

In Chapter 4, "Understanding Oral Diseases: Exploring Opportunities from Filipino Oral Microbiome Research," Prof. Dr. Marilen P. Balolong and Prof. Dr. Michael Antonio F. Mendoza examine the role of oral microbiomes in the human microbial community and human health. Recent advances in technology are slowly revealing the complexity of the oral microbiome, and new insights into its role in health and disease are now being made available. The oral microbiome describes microbial communities' settlement of the oral cavity, which acts as a consortium involved in the modulation of various pathophysiological conditions of the host. It is considered the second most complex in the human body. In addition, the salivary or oral microbiome is the target of interest for diagnostic and prognostic value. Effective preventive measures, accurate diagnosis, sound treatment, and maintenance of good oral health can reduce the global burden of non-communicable diseases such as heart disease and diabetes mellitus. Research and knowledge about the oral microbiome go beyond oral health to the general well-being of individuals and the greater population.

In Chapter 5, "The Application of Fluoride in Dental Caries," Haiyang Sun, Feng Luo, and Qianbing Wan describe the mechanism of fluorides in preventing caries, reducing demineralization, and promoting enamel remineralization. The authors give information about the use of fluoride dental products to prevent cavities. Fluorides can reduce the demineralization of tooth enamel and promote its remineralization. The authors also discuss the different routes of fluoride administration, including fluoride toothpaste, fluoride varnish, fluoride gel, and mouthwash. In some countries, fluoride is added to water, salt, or milk. The authors point out that excessive fluoride intake can cause toxic reactions; tooth fluorosis is caused by high fluoride intake during tooth development. The chapter ends with recommendations for professional topical fluoride application.

In Chapter 6, "The Use of Silver Diamine Fluoride in Pediatric Dentistry," Prof. Dr. Ana Claudia Rodrigues Chibinski provides information about the use of silver diamine fluoride (SDF) in pediatric dentistry. The author presents the composition and mechanism of action of SDF as well as techniques and indications for its application. The effectiveness of SDF is reported based on contemporary scientific evidence from laboratory and clinical studies, focusing on its effect in enamel and dentin remineralization and caries arrestment. The author provides clear information about the use of SDF, indications, advantages, and disadvantages. The low cost and simplicity of the treatment make the use of SDF an interesting option to provide oral care for vulnerable populations without regular access to dental health professionals or in public health dentistry. SDF reduces the growth of cariogenic bacteria, hampers the degradation of collagen in dentin, inhibits demineralization, and promotes remineralization of both enamel and dentin. SDF is a simple and effective treatment to halt dental caries progress in children.

Finally, in Chapter 7, "Caries Experience and Oral Disorders of Disabled Children," Dr. Kuter discusses oral health problems in disabled children who commonly have poor oral healthcare and a high prevalence of caries compared to healthy children. These children often are not able to clarify pain and require special attention from dentists, their parents, and caregivers. This chapter focuses on intraoral manifestations in disabled children with conditions such as Down syndrome, autism, and cerebral palsy. The author elaborates on dental conditions and problems that are more common in children with disabilities, which are due both to mental disability and insufficient oral health care. The author provides clear information from the literature about these patients and the protection of their general and dental health. The information provided should help more dental professionals feel that they have the power to advocate for this patient population.

I acknowledge the desire of the authors who contributed to this important book to share their knowledge with the public. As a professor of Pediatric and Preventive Dentistry, I am especially pleased that dental students at all levels will read this book and learn about the etiology of dental caries as well as preventive measures, especially for patients with disabilities. As a comprehensive and up-to-date summary of the current thinking in the field, this volume is essential reading for not only dental students but also researchers and dental practitioners.

I hope that the scientific evidence and experience presented in this book will enable dental providers to perform evidence-based dental care within the field of cariology and preventive dentistry.

Once again, I would like to thank my colleagues for their contributions to this book.

Dr. Efka Zabokova Bilbilova
Associate Professor,
Department of Pediatric and Preventive Dentistry,
Faculty of Dentistry,
"Ss. Cyril and Methodius" University,
Skopje, Republic of Macedonia

Acknowledgements

To my dear husband Vladimir and my loving son Andrej for their unconditional love and support. I couldn't have made this journey without you. Thank you!

Chapter 1

Introductory Chapter: Dental Biofilms Associated with Caries

Emilija Stefanovska and Efka Zabokova Bilbilova

1. Introduction

Caries is a localized, progressive, destructive process in which the mineral component of dental hard tissues dissolves. It is the result of multiple disturbances of the balance between the oral environment and the teeth. Due to this disturbed balance, microbial acid production occurs and the pH value decreases.

Dental caries is still the most common chronic infectious disease, especially in endangered and poor populations [1, 2], but not so prevalent in the industrialized world and developing countries. Dental caries is a disease associated with biofilm. Plaque control is an important caries prevention strategy, because biofilm bacteria are the driving force of demineralization and caries development [3, 4].

The course of dental caries development depends on several host factors, including location, morphology, composition, ultrastructure, and age of the tooth after eruption [5]. The very environmental conditions that exist at each site of the tooth explain the highly localized and complex nature of the caries process. The occlusal pits and cracks of the molars with their morphological characteristics create a retention area for the formation of biofilm and food retention, making them more prone to caries forming on the tooth surface in children.

The process of dental caries begins within the bacterial biofilm that covers the surface of the tooth. Numerous episodes of mineral loss and gain (demineralization and remineralization) occur on the enamel surface. If demineralization prevails over remineralization, the result will be a permanent and irreversible mineral loss, void formation, and continuous destruction of hard tissues [6, 7]. Signs and symptoms of the disease range from the slightest underground loss of minerals to severe tooth destruction.

Clinical causes of caries include:

1. the presence of plaque containing acid-producing bacteria,

2. consuming carbohydrates that are easily fermented on a frequent basis (for example, sugar),

3. low saliva production or reduced saliva capacity to act as a buffer and.

4. genetic factors which make the host more susceptible to caries [8].

2. Components of dental plaques

The oral microbiome, the unique natural ecology of the mouth is an ecosystem or community of microorganisms that live in symbiosis with one another and with their host, which contribute positively to the individual's health. It is composed of many different bacteria, neutrophils leukocytes, macrophages, monocytes and lymphocytes. The largest portion of dental plaque is liquid and consists of water while 70% of the dry weight is made up of bacteria and the rest is polysaccharide and glycoprotein matrix adherent to the tooth surface [9].

Polysaccharide and glycoprotein matrix mainly consist of 10–20% water-insoluble glucan, 1–2% fructan, approximately 40% bacterial and salivary proteins, variable quantities of lipid, calcium, phosphorus, magnesium and fluoride – the rest is water. The remaining microorganisms are later colonizers that join in the dental biofilm and with their metabolic activities have a competitive advantage in the community [10].

The dental bio-plaque formation is a complex structure, with a highly organized setting of functional symbiotic interactions between microorganisms [11].

The maintenance of health is closely dependent on the balance between the microorganisms that practice commensalism or mutualism between themselves and in relation to the host.

In addition to these interactions, under the influence of certain circumstances, internal or external, this homeostasis may be disturbed, resulting in changes in the microbial population and the induction of certain pathological conditions. An elevation or a depression in the relative presence of certain microorganisms often leads to disruption of homeostasis [12].

A common feature that can disrupt the microbial ecosystem is the import of nutrients, such as sugars. Carbohydrates induce the reproduction of microorganisms that ferment sugars, such as Streptococcus mutans and lactobacilli species. Through metabolizing these carbohydrates, the bacteria generate large amounts of lactic acid, resulting in the selection and dominance of acidogenic bacteria.

The acidogenic oral bacteria present in the dental biofilm, have the ability to generate acids, which are responsible for tooth structure demineralization. The biofilm, related to dental caries, functions in several ways. It is a result of bacterial proliferation and growth, acid/ base regulation at the tooth surface, and a calcium ion exchange between the tooth and the saliva [13].

Many studies have confirmed the role of Streptococcus mutans and some anaerobic bacteria like Fusobacterium and Actinobacilus as a primary colonizer in the initial attachment on the tooth surface, responsible for the formation of the premature biofilm community [14].

The composition of bacterial species like Streptococcus mutans and some anaerobes like Fusobacterium and Actinobacteria varies in the different areas in the mouth. In accordance with the condition and localization of biofilm in the oral cavity there are subclasses of biofilm, sub gingival and supra gingival dental biofilm. Supra gingival plaque usually comprises of aerobic bacteria, thus it is filled with oxygen. On the other hand, sub gingival plaque found in interdental spaces which are devoid of oxygen, consists of anaerobic bacteria.

Changing the conditions in the environment, pH levels, salivary flow, temperature, oxidation–reduction reactions, the growth and development of microorganisms also changes [15]. The normal pH value in the oral cavity varies from 6 to 7. Small deviations from these salivary pH values are a gateway for the multiplication and growth of pathogenic microorganisms, thereby changing the dental plaque formation. The various nutrients in saliva such as proteins and amino acids are an excellent breeding ground for bacterial growth [16]. Deviations from the normal temperature in the oral cavity ranging between 35 and 36 degrees also alter the chemical processes that affect bacterial metabolism. Such a persistent acidic environment within the biofilm results in the demineralization of tooth enamel [17].

However, it should be pointed that streptococcal mutans that produce glucans and biofilm are the primary and major etiological factors in the pathogenesis of dental caries [18].

3. The role of sucrose in biofilm cariogenicity

Numerous epidemiological and experimental studies confirm the causal relationship between sucrose and dental caries [19–22].

Sucrose causes an increased level of Streptococcus mutans and Lactobacilli and at the same time, a decrease in S. sanguinis levels thus leading to biochemical and physiological changes in the dental biofilm formation and enhancing their caries-inducing properties [23]. The cariogenic effect of sucrose is closely dependent on its concentration and duration of exposure [24, 25].

Increasing the frequency of carbohydrates results in plaque accumulation whose persistence below critical pH values will cause demineralization of the enamel [26]. Compared to glucose and fructose, sucrose has the dominant cariogenic potential [27]. As a substrate for the production of extracellular glucan by Streptococcus mutans glycosyltransferases, sucrose takes precedence as a unique cariogenic carbohydrate [28].

4. Dental plaque, a trigger factor in the development of caries and periodontal disease

Scientific research cannot definitively define the concept of a basic, normal oral microbiome that could be associated with a healthy oral cavity for a number of reasons. First of all, because individual dental biofilms are unique, with varying susceptibility to disease. Then with the passage of time and the aging process, the microbial community changes as a result of the evolutionary processes, the ecological environment and the immune response of the individual. However, Gram-positive microorganisms belonging to the streptococcus and actinomyces species are predominantly present in the oral microbiome with certain deviations.

When the transformation of the healthy microbiological community begins and caries occurs, changes in the oral microbiological environment happen, along with changes in the development of the disease [29].

The acidogenic properties of cariogenic microorganisms and the ability to form extracellular polysaccharides from sucrose maintain the acidity of the environment, thus reducing the diversity of microbial flora.

The acidogenic capacity of these microorganisms is the mechanism that is scientifically widely accepted in the process of demineralization of dentinal and enamel tooth structures, causing the development of carious lesions [30].

Dysbiosis in periodontal diseases is also associated with an increase in microbial diversity. The main pathogens in periodontal diseases consist of dominantly gram-negative microorganisms including Porphyromonas gingivalis, Treponema denticola, Tannerella forsythia and Aggregatibacter actinomycetemcomitans [31].

The periodontal microbial community, as dominant in anaerobic conditions, is capable of disrupting the host's inflammatory response by causing nutritional imbalance and impaired availability of potential gingival fluid and blood substrates. The microbial communities in periodontal disease and caries are in symbiosis with the host. How this balance is maintained depends on the nutritional interdependence of the bacteria as well as the salivary glycoproteins which are a constant nutrient source of dental biofilms [29].

The scientific advances in molecular biology have shed light on the bacterial communities present in the oral cavity, providing evidence that the prevalence of oral infections is due to impaired host homeostasis [32–34].

5. Dental indices

Dental indices are a numerical expression for assessing the prevalence and incidence of certain dental conditions, and for determining the need for treatment as well. They can be simple and cumulative. The simple indices determine only the presence or absence of a certain state, while the cumulative ones determine the current state, but also previous, past states. There are also so-called irreversible indices, which determine immutable conditions, such as caries. Reversible indices, in turn, note changing conditions, such as the amount of dental plaque accumulation.

5.1 Oral hygiene index (OHI)

Proposed and developed by John C. Greene and Jack R. Vermillion (1960), [35]. This index is composed of Debris and Calculus Index. Rules for scoring are: 1) Only permanent teeth are scored, 2) Third molars or incompletely erupted teeth are not scored, 3) The buccal and lingual debris scores are both taken on the tooth in a segment having the largest surface area covered by debris. 4) Interpretation: The minimum number of points for all segments in either debris or calculus score is 0. The maximum number of points for all segments in either debris or calculus score is 36. The higher the score, the poorer the oral hygiene.

5.2 Simplified oral hygiene index (OHI-S)

This index is a modification of the original OHI index, also developed by John C. Green and Jack R. Vermillion (1964), [35], in order to reduce the number of decisions made by researches, as well as to shorten the time of inspection. Unlike the original OHI index, rules for scoring are at least two of the six possible tooth surfaces which must be examined. The third molars are involved only as long as they are functional. Natural teeth with crown restorations and tooth surfaces reduced in height by caries or trauma are not recorded.

5.3 Plaque index (PI)

The PI as developed by Silness and Loe [36], assesses the thickness of plaque at the cervical margin of the tooth (closest to the gum). Four areas, distal, facial or buccal, mesial, and lingual, are examined. Each tooth surface should be well dried beforehand, and the examinations are performed with a dental mirror, an explorer and a well-light probe. The probe is passed around the cervical third of the tooth to detect the presence of dental plaque. A disclosing agent can also be used to visualize dental plaque. The results are expressed in four values. A zero indicates no plaque present; 1 indicates a film of plaque present on the tooth; 2 represents moderate accumulation of soft deposits in the gingival pocket or on the tooth that can be seen by the naked eye; 3 represents an abundance of soft matter within the pocket or on the tooth. Each area of each tooth is assigned a score from 0 to 3. Scores for each tooth are totaled and divided by the four surfaces scored. To determine a total PI for an individual, the scores for each tooth are totaled and divided by the number of teeth examined. Four ratings may then be assigned: 0 = excellent, 0.1–0.9 = good, 1.0–1.9 = fair, 2.0–3.0 = poor.

5.4 Gingival index (GI)

Also attributed to Loe and Silness [37], the GI assesses the severity of gingivitis based on color, consistency, and bleeding on probing. Each tooth is examined at the mesial, lingual, distal, and facial (or buccal) surface. A probe is used to press on the gingiva to determine its degree of firmness, and to run along the soft tissue wall adjacent to the entrance to the gingival sulcus. Four criteria are possible: 0, normal gingiva; 1, mild inflammation but no bleeding on probing; 2, moderate inflammation and bleeding on probing; 3, severe inflammation and ulceration, with a tendency for spontaneous bleeding. Each surface is given a score, then the scores are totaled and divided by four. That number is divided by the number of teeth examined to determine the GI. Ratings are 0 = excellent; 0.1–1.0 = good; 1.1–2.0 = fair; 2.1–3.0 = poor.

6. Conclusion

Dental biofilm, as a proven complex biostructure of microorganisms is the primary etiological factor for the development of the two most diseases in the oral cavity - caries and periodontal diseases. Despite the fact that it cannot be completely eradicated, it can be controlled. So, the risk assessment for its occurrence is essential for the preservation of oral health. An individual adaptive anti-plaque program should be applied to each patient with a recommendation for appropriate home oral hygiene, practicing daily tooth brushing with a fluoride tooth paste, interdental cleaning and a hygienic-diet regimen with reduced carbohydrate intake. By doing this, there is an optimistic possibility that these cost-effective preventive strategies may minimize the incidence of caries and periodontal diseases and their impact on specific systemic conditions.

Author details

Emilija Stefanovska* and Efka Zabokova Bilbilova
Department of Periodontology and Oral Medicine, Faculty of Dentistry, "Ss. Cyril and Methodius" University, Skopje, Republic of Macedonia

*Address all correspondence to: emistefanovska@yahoo.com

References

[1] Dantas Cabral de Melo MM, de Souza WV, Tavares MC, de Lima ML, Jamelli S, Couto GB. Social conditions and high levels of dental caries in five-year-old children in Brazil. J Dent Child (Chic) 2015; 82:29-35.

[2] Sinha N, Singh B, Chhabra KG, Patil Comparison of oral health status between children with cerebral palsy and normal children in India: a case-control study. J Indian Soc Periodontol 2015;19: 78-82.

[3] Takahashi N, Nyvad B. Caries ecology revisited: microbial dynamics and the caries process. Caries Res 2008 42, 409-418.

[4] Ccahuana-Vásquez RA, Cury JA. S. mutans biofilm model to evaluate antimicrobial substances and enamel demineralization. Braz Oral Res 2010; 24: 135-141.

[5] Guido JA, Martinez Mier EA, Soto A, Eggertsson H, Sanders BJ, Jones JE, Weddell JA, Villanueva Cruz I, de la Concha A, Luis J. Caries prevalence and its association with brushing habits, water availability, and the intake of sugared beverages. International Journal of Paediatric Dentistry 2011;21(6):432-440.

[6] Caufield PW, Li Y, Dasanayake A. Dental caries: an infectious and transmissible disease. Compend Contin Educ Dent 2005; 26 (5 Suppl 1):10-6.

[7] Takahashi N, Nyvad B. The role of bacteria in the caries process: ecological perspectives. J Dent Res 2011; 90: 294-303.

[8] Kutsch VK. Dental caries: an updated medical model of risk assessment. J Prosthet Dent 2014; 111: 2805.

[9] Marsh PD, Moter A, Devine DA. Dental plaque biofilms: communities, conflict and control. Periodontol 2000 2011; 55:16-35.

[10] Bowen WH, Koo H. Biology of Streptococcus mutans-derived glucosyltransferases: role in extracellular matrix formation of cariogenic biofi lms. Caries Res 2011; 45:69-86.

[11] Marsh PD, Bradshaw DJ. "Dental plaque as a biofilm". J Ind Microbiol 1995; 15(3): 169-175.

[12] Kolenbrander PE. "Oral Microbial Communities: Biofilms, Interactions, and Genetic Systems". Annu Rev Microbiol 2000; 54(1):413-437.

[13] Bradshaw DJ, McKee AS, Marsh PD. Effects of carbohydrate pulses and pH on population shifts within oral microbial communities in vitro. J Dent Res 1989; 68(9):1298-302.13.

[14] Chetrus V, Ion IR. "Dental Plaque - Classification, Formation, and Identification." Int J Med Dentistry 2013; 3(2):139-143.

[15] Mc Dermid AS, McKee AS, Marsh PD. "Effect of Environmental pH on Enzyme Activity and Growth of Bacteroides gingival is W50". Infect Immun 1998; 56(5): 1096-100.

[16] Humphrey SP, Williamson RT. A review of saliva: normal composition, flow, and function J Prosthet Dent 2011 85(2): 162-169.

[17] Marsh PD, Devine DA (2011) "How is the development of dental biofilms influenced by the host?" J Clin Periodontol 38 (s11): 28-35.

[18] Zhou M, Zhu F, Dong S, Pritchard D, Wu H. A novel glucosyltransferase is required for glycosylation of a serine-rich adhesin and biofilm formation by Streptococcus parasanguinis. J Biol Chem 2010; 285:12140-8.

[19] Cury JA, Rebelo MA, Del Bel Cury AA, Derbyshire MT, Tabchoury CP. Biochemical composition and cariogenicity of dental plaque formed in the presence of sucrose or glucose and fructose. Caries Res 2000; 34:491-497.

[20] Cury JA, Francisco SB, Del Bel Cury AA, Tabchoury CP. In situ study of sucrose exposure, mutans streptococci in dental plaque and dental caries. Braz Dent J 2001; 12:101-104.

[21] Cury JA, Marques AS, Tabchoury CP, Del Bel Cury AA. Composition of dental plaque formed in the presence of sucrose and after its interruption. Braz Dent J 2003; 14:147-152.

[22] Zero DT. Sugars-the arch criminal? Caries Res 2004; 38:277-285.

[23] Minah GE, Lovekin GB, Finney JP. Sucrose-induced ecological response of experimental dental plaques from caries-free and caries-susceptible human volunteers. Infect Immun 1981; 34:662-675.

[24] Aires CP, Tabchoury CP, Del Bel Cury AA, Koo H, Cury JA. Effect of sucrose concentration on dental biofilm formed in situ and on enamel demineralization. Caries Res 2006; 40:28-32.

[25] Paes Leme AF, Dalcico R, Tabchoury CP, Del Bel Cury AA, Rosalen PL, Cury JA. In situ effect of frequent sucrose exposure on enamel demineralization and on plaque composition after APF application and F dentifrice use. J Dent Res 2004; 83:71-75.

[26] Marsh PD. Sugar, fluoride, pH and microbial homeostasis in dental plaque. Proc Finn Dent Soc 1991; 87:515-525.

[27] Cury JA, Rebelo MA, Del Bel Cury AA, Derbyshire MT, Tabchoury CP. Biochemical composition and cariogenicity of dental plaque formed in the presence of sucrose or glucose and fructose. Caries Res 2000; 34:491-497

[28] Bowen WH. Do we need to be concerned about dental caries in the coming millennium? Crit Rev Oral Biol Med 2002; 13:126-131.

[29] Mira A, Simon-Soro A & Curtis MA. Role of microbial communities in the pathogenesis of periodontitis and caries. Journal of Clinical Periodontology 2017; 44: S18, 23-38.

[30] Simón-Soro A & Mira A. Solving the etiology of dental caries. Trends in Microbiology 2015; 23:76-82.

[31] Camelo-Castillo AJ, Mira A, Pico A, Nibali L, Henderson B, Donos N & Tomás I. Subgingival microbiota in health compared to periodontitis and the influence of smoking. Frontiers in Microbiology 2015; 24:119.

[32] Darveau RP. Periodontitis: a polymicrobial disruption of host homeostasis. Nat Rev Microbiol 2010; 8(7):481-490.

[33] Kuramitsu HK, He X, Lux R, et al. Interspecies interactions within oral microbial communities. Microbiol Mol Biol Rev 2007; 71(4):653-670.

[34] Von Fraunhofer JA, Loewy ZG (2009) Factors involved in microbial colonization of oral prostheses. Gen Dent 57(2): 136-143.

[35] Greene JC. and Vermillion JR. The Simplified Oral Hygiene Index. The Journal of the American Dental Association 1964; 68:7-13.

[36] Silness P, Löe H. Periodontal disease in pregnancy II. Acta Odontol Scand. 1964; 22:121-6.

[37] Löe H, Silness P. Periodontal disease in pregnancy I. Acta Odontol Scand 1963; 21:533-51.

Chapter 2

Dietary Factors, Salivary Parameters, and Dental Caries

Efka Zabokova Bilbilova

Abstract

Diet and oral microflora are connected to caries along with host factors such as salivary composition and flow. The only component of the food with potentially cariogenic effect is fermentable carbohydrate sucrose. Sucrose is generally accepted as the most cariogenic dietary factor, and consumption of sucrose is associated with the frequency of dental caries in humans. Saliva is a biological environment, important for the physiology of the mouth. It achieves its mechanical functions of cleaning and protection through various physical and biochemical mechanisms. Bicarbonates, phosphates, and proteins have a buffer role in the saliva environment. Other compounds or enzymes in this group acting as prophylactic buffers are urea, salivary amylases, and fluorides.

Keywords: dental caries, diet, sucrose, saliva, salivary buffer

1. Introduction

From the ancient time, dental caries has existed, even from the time when the only way to eat and drink was hunting and gathering. According to the World Health Organization, 60–90% of schoolchildren worldwide have experienced caries, with the disease being most prevalent in Asian and Latin American countries (WHO, 2008). Dental caries is a multifactor disease which appears when demineralization of the hard tissues of the teeth occurs by organic acids formed by bacteria in dental plaque through the anaerobic metabolism of sugars derived from the diet.

Calcium is lost from the tooth surface, and demineralization occurs only when sugars or other fermentable carbohydrates are ingested in which results fall in dental plaque pH caused by organic acids that increase the solubility of calcium hydroxyapatite in the dental hard tissues.

Lifestyle or dental health habits are the factors that should be connected to dental diseases. Dietary and daily habits, familial and physiological well-being, socioeconomic status and lifestyle, awareness and education, and area where they live are the factors that should be taken into consideration when discussing oral health. The higher the socioeconomic status is, the more the people are exposed to the availability of junk foods and susceptible to its frequent consumption. Those from lower economic group and rural area are not as much exposed to such food habits, and they do not buy them because they are expensive for their pocket. Many adolescents fail to brush their teeth effectively and tend to consume cariogenic foods even though they have basic knowledge of dental health. Children who have caries eat snacks between meals, more than those children without dental caries do. The basic means of avoiding these primary public health measures are compiled with the use of topical fluorides and fluoridated water. When it comes to nutrition perspective, one of the main things is to have balanced diet and adherence to the dietary guidelines and the dietary reference intakes.

1.1 The dental caries process

Dental caries occurs due to the demineralization of enamel and dentin (the hard tissues of the teeth) by organic acids formed by bacteria in dental plaque through the anaerobic metabolism of sugars and other fermentable carbohydrates derived from the diet [1]. Organic acids increase the solubility of calcium hydroxyapatite in dental hard tissues, and demineralization process of the tooth surface occurs due to calcium loss.

Teeth are most susceptible to dental caries soon after they erupt, and therefore the peak ages for dental caries are 2–5 years for the deciduous dentition and early adolescence for the permanent dentition [2]. The age of adolescences is when permanent teeth begin to grow and get their full position in the dental arch. This is a crucial age for the development of several oral diseases. Dental caries, periodontal disease, and orthodontic problems such as overcrowding of the teeth or malocclusions are bringing changes and altering the facial profile and esthetic appearance.

Certain psychological factors like self-confidence and social outlook of the individuals can also be affected, and they can leave permanent effect on the psychology of the child if not appropriately treated.

Neglecting the general problems, the lack of awareness and expertise is one of the reasons that most of the children at this age face these problems. Since the treatment of dental disease is very expensive especially in low-income countries, it would exceed the available resources for health care. The large financial benefits of preventing dental diseases should be emphasized to countries where current disease levels are high [3].

1.2 Effects of dental caries

It is undisputable that the development of dental caries is a result of poor diet, and it has been observed in humans and animals that frequent and prolonged exposure to carbohydrates and sugars results in an appearance of dental caries. Important bacteria in the development of dental caries are *Streptococcus mutans* and *Streptococcus sobrinus*. These bacteria produce organic acids from food sugars and help bacterial colonization of the tooth surface. The bacteria attached to teeth in dental plaque, found as a thin film on the surface of the enamel, utilize mono- and disaccharides (e.g., glucose, fructose, and sucrose) to produce energy, and acid is the by-product of this metabolism.

Consequently, the acidity of dental plaque may decrease to a point where the demineralization of the tooth begins. Demineralization occurs at a low pH when the oral environment is undersaturated with mineral ions, relative to a tooth's mineral content. The enamel crystal, which consists of carbonated apatite, is dissolved by organic acids (lactic and acetic) that are produced by the cellular action of plaque bacteria in the presence of dietary carbohydrates. The "white spot lesion" is the initial stage that occurs just below the enamel surface and produces a visual whitening of the tooth. At this stage of mineral loss, the lesion may not progress any further or could even regain minerals (i.e., remineralize) if the cariogenic environment diminishes. The prevention measures that can remineralize the initial carious lesion are as follows: decreasing the carbohydrate source to the bacteria, treating the tooth with fluoride, reducing the levels of cariogenic bacteria, or reducing the bacterial ability to produce acid.

The initial lesion will continue to lose mineral if the procedure of disease suppression is not initiated and the acidic challenge is unabated. The progressive dissolution of enamel and loss of enamel surface structure eventually give rise to a frank carious lesion [4]. Sugary food products and their everyday consumptions exert our teeth. The reasons behind dental caries are the exposure to junk foods, colas, sweets, and other dietary products which are easy to access and abundantly available for children to consume. That is why dental caries is like a sort of non-transmittable and nonfatal sickness [5].

1.3 Dietary factors in the initiation and progression of dental caries

Some authors emphasize the importance of the dental biofilm and dietary sugars as essential primary etiological factors causing the appearance of the caries; moreover, one of them cannot cause caries in the absence of the other.

The main direct impact of the diet is mediated through its effect on the pH of the dental biofilm. Foods high in fermentable carbohydrates (mainly sugars) cause a low biofilm pH, while foods high in proteins and fats favor a more neutral biofilm pH. High-protein foods increase the urea concentration of saliva, which can be converted by ureolytic bacteria to ammonia; this raises the biofilm pH and is associated with decreased caries risk. Dietary factors can have an indirect effect by modifying the composition and metabolic activity of dental biofilm.

The major dietary factor affecting dental caries prevalence and progression is sucrose [6]. A low consumption example is from a study of the Hopewood House in Australia, conducted between 1947 and 1952. As a matter of fact, children living in this closely supervised environment consumed food that was virtually free of sugar and white flour products. Data collected from these children revealed an extremely low dental caries prevalence, compared to children attending other Australian schools [7].

High sugar consumption's effect is best revealed from the report of the classic Vipeholm study [8]. This study examined three factors leading to these stages as follows: the timing of sugar ingestion, the effects of the frequency of sugar consumption, and finally the consistency of the sugar on dental caries rates. According to the results, the degree of the sugar's consistency was more important than the addition of sugar to the diet and especially if it was consumed between meals, or products, which are sticky, in a form that stayed longer in the mouth such as toffees. These products have a bigger cariogenicity impact than foods that are eliminated quickly from the oral cavity. Therefore, frequent ingestion of foods such as hard candies and throat lozenges that contain fermentable carbohydrates can be extremely harmful to the teeth. The conclusions from this study, conducted a half century ago, are still well regarded today:

1. If sugar is taken with meals, then only a small caries increase is noted.

2. A marked increase in caries increment is shown if sugar is consumed as snacks between meals.

3. If you consume sticky candies containing sugar, then the caries activity will be at the highest form.

4. Caries activity may vary greatly among individuals.

5. By eliminating sugar-rich foods, caries activity will be declined.

The detrimental effects of sugar in causing tooth decay are shown in the two major studies of public health importance, and those are the classic Vipeholm study in Sweden and Hopewood House study in Australia. Children generally consume diets which are rich in sugar like sweets, candies, cakes, colas, etc. That is why a lot of awareness has been raised since this food has a negative effect on oral health, and that is the appearance of dental caries. Nowadays, the household food that we generally eat contains certain amounts of sugar. That is why these two studies are of huge public health importance when conducting preventive dental health programs especially in schools where the drawbacks of consuming such diet containing sugars can be addressed.

1.4 Food products that play a main role in the development of dental caries

A direct relationship between dental caries incidence and sugar (carbohydrates) intake is indisputed. The caries will not be developed if there are no fermentable carbohydrates in the food [9].

Free sugars as defined by the World Health Organization present as monosaccharides and disaccharides added to food, and sugars are naturally present in honey, syrups, and fruit juices. Fermentable carbohydrates are free sugars, glucose polymers (syrups and maltodextrins), fermentable oligosaccharides, and highly refined starches. They are added to food in industrialized countries and are as acidogenic as sucrose. However, sucrose and starches today present as the main carbohydrates in modern society diet. Sucrose is the most cariogenic sugar which is a highly soluble substrate transformed into intracellular (IPS) and extracellular polysaccharides (EPS). It diffuses easily into the dental plaque accumulation and induces a lower pH [10]. **Starch** is a carbohydrate that can cause very small amounts of caries, unlike real sugar. It is found in fruits and vegetables and can be consumed raw or cooked. Starchy foods such as rice, potatoes, pasta, and bread have very low cariogenicity, and this is why they can cause less caries than sucrose. Starch can be sorted out to mono- and disaccharides and metabolized by bacteria, so it is retained on the teeth long enough to be hydrolyzed by salivary amylase.

Since the original Miller's study, Stephan in both of his researches (1940, 1944) about the relationship between caries and sugar showed that fermentable carbohydrates can transform into acid in dental plaque. A direct relationship between caries incidence and the frequency of consumption of sweets was also presented [11], and these findings supported those of the Vipeholm study [12].

Sucrose is freely diffusible in dental biofilm and metabolized by oral bacteria *Streptococcus mutans* [13]. Bacteria metabolize sucrose to soluble and insoluble extracellular polysaccharide glucan by enzyme glucosyltransferases (GTFs). Few mechanisms are involved in the role of extracellular glucans as the major caries associated factor. Glucan enables the bacteria to adhere firmly to the teeth [14], and in dental plaque, they contribute to the structural integrity of dental biofilms [15].

Several studies showed that the presence of insoluble glucan enhanced the demineralization potential of *S. mutans*. Glucan altered the diffusion properties of plaque and allowed deeper penetration of dietary carbohydrates [16, 17].

There are several important and critical cariogenic factors to be considered when evaluating starch and caries relationship. They are the size and frequency of tooth exposure, the bioavailability of the starches, the microbial flora of dental plaque, the pH-lowering capacity of dental plaque, and the flow rate of saliva. Starchy foods with higher amounts of sucrose are as cariogenic as a sucrose. Some cooked and processed starches are dissolved by salivary amylase, and they release glucose and maltose metabolized by oral bacteria to acids. In Rugg-Gunn [18] study, the relationship between starches and dental caries was proved, and several conclusions were made. Rice, potatoes, bread, and cooked staple starchy foods have low cariogenicity in humans. Uncooked starch has low cariogenicity, while heat-treated starch induces lesser caries than sugars. Foods with cooked starch and higher amounts of sucrose are as cariogenic as similar quantities of sucrose.

Fresh fruits contain various sugars and may be capable of causing caries under some conditions. They have low cariogenicity, while citrus fruits have not been associated with dental caries. Increased consumption of fresh fruit in the diet is decreasing the level of dental caries in a population [19]. Although excessive exposure to fructose may produce dental caries, fresh fruits are likely to be much less cariogenic than most sucrose-rich snack foods consumed by children. One hundred percent fruit juice has also been associated with caries, but the relationship is less clear. Children consuming more than 17 oz. 100% juice are more likely to have caries, than children consuming water or milk [20]. Conversely, in a cohort of low-income African-American children, 100% fruit juice was found to be protective of caries. The fact that 100% fruit juice contains about the same amount of sugar as the average sugar-sweetened beverages made it important to understand its role in caries [21]. Animal studies revealed that all fruits cause less caries than sucrose but dried fruits may potentially be more cariogenic since the drying process breaks down the cellular structure, releasing free sugars that tend to have a longer oral clearance.

Flavored drinks, especially aerated beverages like cola, have a much greater cariogenic potential due to high sugar content and regular consumption. Children are frequently offered with these drinks because of their high acceptance, low cost, and parent's belief of being very nutritious [22]. Different campaigns and various forms of advertising by the media changed public health knowledge, and people started to become aware and understand about the bad effect of this kind of food.

Milk is most frequently consumed by schoolchildren. In milk a sugar named lactose is not fermented as the other sugars, so it is less cariogenic because the phosphor proteins inhibit enamel dissolution and the milk antibacterial factors may interfere with the oral microbial flora.

Cheese can lead to protection against creating caries as it stimulates salivary flow and raises the calcium, phosphorus, and protein content of plaque.

The sugar alcohols like sorbitol, mannitol, and xylitol are kind of sweeteners that are metabolized by bacteria at much slower rate than glucose or sucrose, which is not metabolized at all. According to certain clinical studies, xylitol chewing gum has the ability to reverse initial white spot lesions on teeth.

When dental decay happens there is high probability of losing a tooth. That leads to a reduced ability to eat a varied diet. It is in particular associated with a low consumption of fruits, vegetables and non-starch polysaccharides (NSP) in the persons diet [23]. NSP intakes of less than 10 g/day and fruits and vegetable intakes of less than 160 g/day have been reported in edentulous subjects. Therefore, tooth loss may impede the achievement of dietary goals related to the consumption of fruits, vegetables, and NSP. Tooth loss has also been associated with loss of enjoyment of food and confidence to socialize. So, basically, it is clear that dental diseases have a detrimental effect on the quality of life both in childhood and older age [24].

1.5 Eating between meals

An important issue for the appearance of dental caries in older children as well as infants is not only the total quantity but also the form of the carbohydrate as well as the frequency of consumption since the refined carbohydrates exert their effect in the appearance of dental caries by serving as a substrate for caries-producing streptococci, which as a small piece of it adheres to the teeth for almost an hour. In the case of sugars that are not in sticky form, a specified amount consumed at one time is likely to be less conducive to the formation of dental caries than the same amount consumed in small portions throughout the day. There is considerable evidence that between-meal snacks cause the development of dental caries. Foods that must be avoided between meals are the following: sugar, honey, corn syrup, candies, jellies, jams, sugared breakfast cereals, cookies, cakes, chewing gum, and sweetened beverages, including flavored kind of milks, carbonated drinks, sweetened fruit juices, and fruit or fruit-flavored drinks. Finally, eating frequency, particularly constant grazing or sipping of foods and beverages, is also caries promoting. In a recent study in a diverse sample of children aged 2 to 6 years, eating frequency was associated with severe early childhood caries [25].

1.6 Dietary fluoride and water fluoridation

Reduction of dental caries can be achieved with the help of fluoride or in other words dietary fluoride drinking water, which also has rich sources. The ingested fluoride becomes incorporated into enamel during tooth formation and increases the resistance of the tooth to decay. However, the main protection from dietary fluoride is the localized intraoral effect. Fluoride promotes the remineralization of damaged enamel with resistant fluorapatite and also inhibits bacterial metabolism of sugars. As we can see, the benefits to the exposure of teeth to fluoride are therefore beneficial lifelong. It may be added to an optimum concentration of 1 mg/L as a caries preventive measure if natural water supplies are low in fluoride; Murray et al. [26] have reviewed the published data on the effect of water fluoridation on caries and have concluded that on average water fluoridation reduces dental caries by 50%. In a study of 5-year-old children, Carmichael et al. have demonstrated that water fluoridation is effective in reducing dental caries across social classes and, in terms of the number of teeth saved per child, the benefits are greatest in the lower social classes [27].

According to UK national surveys, it has been indicated that those from lower social classes have higher levels of dental diseases and poorer oral hygiene practice and are less likely to visit the dentist [28]. In these cases, dental caries is not eliminated even though the benefit of fluoride is reducing caries. Fluoride repairs the damage caused by acids produced by plaque bacteria but does not remove the cause of caries, i.e., dietary sugars. The process of prevention requires both a reduction in sugar intake as well as optimum exposure to fluoride. Very extensive and comprehensive research by the National Health Survey concluded that a preventive dentistry program is water fluoridation.

1.7 Dietary advice

Dietary advice by dental health professionals should be consistent and not conflict with the advices from other health professionals, based on the evidence in the various professional fields and based on the national dietary guidelines. The advices may be more readily accepted from the people when the oral healthcare professionals can make unequivocally clear that the advice benefits caries prevention. If not, the person may not understand why the dental professional interferes with his diet and not accept the advices. However, this does not dismiss the dental professional from also explaining the benefits for general health on limiting or reducing the intake of sugars. Under the premise that it benefits oral health, the dental health professional can make stronger restrictions than the general guidelines as long as they do not harm general health. Generally speaking a diet that is beneficial to both general and dental health is one that is low in free sugars, saturated fat, and salts, as well as high in fresh fruits, vegetables, nuts and seeds, and wholegrain carbohydrates with modest amounts of legumes, fish, poultry, and lean meat and plenty of fluids preferably water and milk and, thus, modest with sugar sweetened beverages [29].

2. Saliva and oral health

The teeth and oral mucosa are cleaned with the help of saliva, which is a mixed glandular secretion. Saliva by itself is consisted of three glands, and they are as follows: submandibular, sublingual, and finally the parotid. It also has hundreds of small glands inside the oral mucosa and submucosa as well as gingival cervical fluid.

The maintenance of healthy teeth and oral tissues could be achieved only with the help of saliva's presence. If there were a severe reduction of the saliva's production, then there would be a very fast deterioration of oral health as well as the patient's life. The results from such a condition could lead to eating difficulties like: swallowing difficulties, bad oral hygiene, dental caries that progresses very fast, mucosa's burning sensation, difficulty in talking, wearing denture, oral infections like *Candida*, and ulceration of oral mucosa.

Dry mouth is a problem, which appears in huge proportions. Xerostomia or in other words dry mouth is very common for people with Sjogren's syndrome, as a result of radiotherapy in the head and neck in cancer treating and especially in the case of older generations when they are prescribed with drugs. The saliva's role in oral health is huge especially taking into consideration the sicknesses that appear because of decreased quantity or quality of saliva. That is why it is very important to early diagnose and prevent this condition.

Saliva is considered as the most easily available diagnostic fluid for noninvasive collection and analysis because through it we can diagnose caries susceptibility, systemic, physiological, and pathological, and we can monitor the level of hormones, drugs, antibodies, microorganisms, and ions.

In this research, we will try to present the main functions of saliva, the anatomy and histology of salivary glands, the physiology of saliva formation, the constituents of saliva, and the use of saliva as a diagnostic fluid, including its role in caries risk assessment.

2.1 Saliva's functions

Saliva has several functions which are very protective, but it has also other functions presented in **Figure 1**. Salivary function can be organized into five major categories that serve to maintain oral health and create an appropriate ecologic balance: (1) lubrication and protection, (2) buffering action and clearance, (3) maintenance of tooth integrity, (4) antibacterial activity, and (5) taste and digestion [30].

Figure 2 presents the changes in plaque pH following as a result of sucrose rinse. The graphs are named as Stephan's curve according to the name of the scientist who was the first one who described it in 1944. By using antimony probe microelectrodes in a series of experiments, he also measured changes in plaque pH.

The unstimulated plaque pH in **Figure 2** is approximately 6.7. After the process of sucrose rinse, the plaque pH within a few minutes is reduced to less than 5.0. When the enamel is below the critical pH 5.5, then there is demineralization of the enamel. For about 15–20 min, plaque pH stays below the critical pH and does return to normal for about 40 min. In the presence of saliva and other fluids that are supersaturated with the help of hydroxyapatite and fluorapatite, the enamel itself could be remineralized only when the plaque pH recovers to a level above the critical pH.

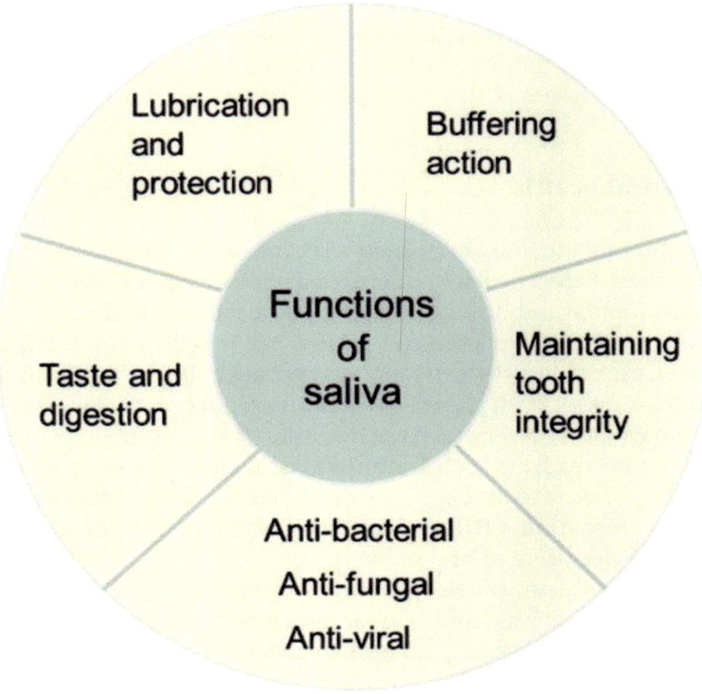

Figure 1.
Functions of saliva.

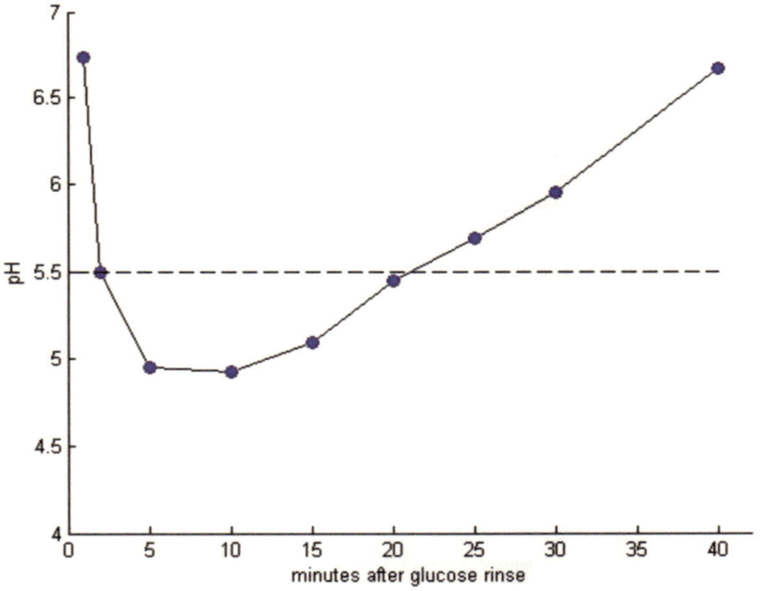

Figure 2.
Stephan's curve illustrating the changes in plague pH over time following a sucrose rinse.

The buffering capacity, the degree of access to saliva, the velocity of the salivary film, and the saliva's urea content are the ones that determine the variation of the shape of Stephan's curve among individuals and the rate of recovery of the pH plaque.

The major buffer in stimulated saliva is the carbonic acid/bicarbonate system. As the bicarbonate ion concentration gets higher, also the buffering capacity of saliva increases.

2.2 Saliva as a diagnostic fluid

2.2.1 General diagnostics

Nowadays for the study of bacteria, proteins, and genes, there are very high-level techniques where they apply saliva in order to spread out the field of oral diagnostics in the process of learning and understanding the oral diseases, systemic diseases, as well as metabolism. Saliva by itself presents an opportunity for the identification of biomarkers for the diseases like dental caries, periodontal diseases, and oral diseases, but all this should be easily done with careful collection and handling.

2.3 Caries risk assessment

There have been developed a series of caries risk assessment tests based on saliva's measurements. These tests measure the capacity of salivary buffering and salivary mutans streptococci and lactobacilli. The increased risk of developing caries comes because of high levels of mutans streptococci, i.e., >105 colony-forming units (CFUs) per mL of saliva. Individuals with high levels of lactobacilli (>105 CFUs per mL saliva) are the ones who consume frequently carbohydrates, and because of that they have an increased risk of caries.

As an answer to the question what is buffering capacity, one could answer that it is the host's capability to neutralize reduction pH's plaque constructed by acidogenic organisms. Useful caries indicators for monitoring, preventive measures, and profiling patient's disease are the salivary tests.

Table 1 lists some salivary variables measured for caries risk assessment in dentistry, which are more used for measurement than the other types.

While either measuring unstimulated or stimulated saliva's flow rates, we should bear in mind the conditions of saliva's collection process. When measuring unstimulated flow, which is usually at rest, repeated measurements should be assessed during the same day as a result of circadian rhythm and also because chewing (mechanical) and citric acid (gustatory) produce different results.

The best way of measuring unstimulated or stimulated saliva is using commercial kit. When it comes to buffering capacity of unstimulated saliva which is lower or stimulated saliva, they are very easily measured at the chairside. In order to do bacteriological tests as chewing dislodges the flora into the saliva, then the best way is to use paraffin wax-stimulated saliva samples. From stimulated saliva samples, you can culture mutans streptococci and lactobacilli. Their measurements could also be facilitated with the help of commercially available chairside tests. However, when it comes to fluoride, calcium, and phosphate biochemical measurement, then these must be done with the help of special laboratory facilities that are not available to practitioners.

2.4 Unstimulated saliva

As an answer to the question what is unstimulated whole saliva, one could answer that it is the mouth's secretion mixture with tastants or chewing in the absence of exogenous stimuli. It is composed of parotid, submandibular, and sublingual secretions as well as the minor mucous glands, but it also contains

Fluid/lubricant	It coats hard and soft tissue. Helps to protect against mechanical, thermal, and chemical irritation and tooth wear. Assists smooth air flow, speech, and swallowing.
Ion reservoir	Solution supersaturated with respect to tooth mineral facilitates remineralization of the teeth. Acidic proline-rich proteins and statherin in saliva inhibit spontaneous precipitation of calcium phosphate salts.
Buffering action and clearance	Helps to neutralize plaque pH after eating, thus reducing time for demineralization.
Mechanical function of cleaning the tooth surface	Clears food and aids swallowing.
Antimicrobial activity	Specific (e.g., sIgA) and non-specific (e.g. lysozyme, lactoferrin, and myeloperoxidase) anti-microbial mechanisms help to control the oral microflora.
Digestion	The enzyme α-amylase is the most abundant salivary enzyme; it splits starchy foods into maltose, maltotriose, and dextrins.
Protective remineralization (promoted by fluoride)	Saliva also inhibits caries by protective remineralization. This is promoted by fluoride ions in saliva.

Table 1.
Salivary variables measured for caries risk assessment.

desquamated epithelial cells, gingival crevicular fluid, leucocytes (mainly from the gingival crevice), bacteria, and possibly food residues, blood, and viruses.

The collection of saliva from the patient is done in that way that the patient spits out saliva in regular intervals of time without swallowing it, and there is another way when the patient keeps his or her head down and mouth just a bit open so that saliva can drip down from the mouth into a beaker during a time interval. However, one should bear in mind that when saliva is spit down, the number of desquamated epithelial cells as well as bacteria are increased. The difference between the secreted amount by the different salivary glands and the evaporated volumes is the measured flow rate. The unstimulated salivary flow rates in healthy individuals and the average value for whole saliva is about 0.3–0.4 mL/min. Patients say that they have dry mouth (xerostomia) only when saliva is almost completely absent. Objective evidence of hyposalivation is considered a flow rate of <0.1 mL/min.

Dentists should also measure salivary flow as part of their regular examination so that when patients complain of dry mouth, they will have the tests. The usual problems are related to swallowing difficulty that often leads to individuals with very little saliva but without discomfort and others with saliva flow rates within the normal range who feel that their mouth is drowning in saliva.

2.5 Stimulated saliva

Stimulated saliva is produced in response to a mechanical, gustatory, olfactory, or pharmacological stimulus, contributing to around 40–50% of daily salivary production. Several studies of stimulated salivary flow rates have been done in healthy populations and show a wide variation among individuals. The salivary flow (SF) index is a parameter allowing stimulated and unstimulated saliva flow to be classified as normal, low, or very low (hyposalivation). In adults, normal total stimulated SF ranges 1–3 mL/min, and low ranges 0.7–1.0 mL/min, while hyposalivation is characterized by a stimulated SF <0.7 mL/min. Many factors influence the stimulated salivary flow rate which, for whole saliva, has an average maximum value of about 7 mL/min.

2.5.1 Mechanical stimuli

Eating is a strong stimulus for the secretion of saliva by the major salivary glands. Large volumes of saliva are secreted before, during, and after eating via the gustatory-salivary reflex, masticatory-salivary reflex, olfactory-salivary reflex, and esophageal-salivary reflex. The action of chewing, in the absence of any taste, will stimulate salivation to a smaller degree than maximum gustatory stimulation with citric acid. Mastication also serves to mix the contents of the mouth, thus increasing slightly the distribution of the different types of saliva around the mouth. Mechanical stimulation of the fauces (the gag reflex) leads to increased salivation.

2.5.2 Gustatory and olfactory stimuli

Acid is the most potent of the five basic taste stimuli, the other four being salty, bitter, sweet, and umami. A study performed with different concentrations of citric acid revealed that 5% citric acid stimulated an average maximum salivary flow rate of about 7 mL/min. The citric acid was continuously infused into the mouth, and the teeth were covered with a paraffin film to protect them against the acid. For a clinical evaluation of the residual secretory capacity in patients with hyposalivation, a 3% citric acid solution can be applied to the patient's tongue at regular intervals so that the degree of stimulation is relatively standardized. If a gustatory stimulus is held in the mouth without movement, salivary flow decreases to nature of stimulus gland size, mechanical unilateral stimulation, gustatory vomiting, pharmacological olfaction, food intake smoking, and gag reflex.

Dawes [31] has stimulated the flow of saliva alters its composition and noted that the rate of salivary flow increases the concentration of protein, sodium, chloride, and bicarbonate and decreases the concentration of magnesium and phosphorus. Perhaps of greatest importance is the increase in the concentration of bicarbonate, which increases progressively with the duration of stimulation. The increased concentration of bicarbonate diffuses into the plaque, neutralizes plaque acids, increases the pH of the plaque, and favors the remineralization of damaged enamel and dentin.

2.6 Saliva's buffering ability

Buffer solutions are solutions that maintain an approximately constant pH when small amounts of either acid or base are added or when the solution is diluted. These solutions own the capacity of resisting changes of pH when either acids or alkalis are added to them. There are three possible buffer systems in saliva—the carbonic acid/bicarbonate system, the phosphate system, and the proteins.

2.6.1 Bicarbonate

Bicarbonate is one of the most important systems in saliva, which is produced by dental plaque, and its concentration could be from less than 1 mmol/L in unstimulated parotid saliva to a very high flow rate of 60 mmol/L which is elicited by chewing gum thus having a bicarbonate concentration of about 15 mmol/L. The level of bicarbonate ions in unstimulated saliva is too low to be an effective buffer. For those who suffer from the gastroesophageal reflux disease, the bicarbonate in saliva will help them in the clearance process of acid from the esophagus.

The carbonic acid/bicarbonate system is one of the components of the saliva that modifies the creation of caries. It does this by changing the environmental pH and possibly the virulence of bacteria that cause decay. Tanzer et al. [32] tasted the efficacy of a sodium bicarbonate-based dental power and paste with the addition of fluoride on dental caries and on *Streptococcus sobrinus* or *Streptococcus mutans* recoveries in rats. These authors observed that the caries reductions in these studies ranged from 42 to 50% in the rats treated with bicarbonate dentifrices when compared with rats treated with water [33, 34].

2.6.2 Phosphate

The concentration of phosphate in non-stimulated saliva is about 5–6 mmol/L, compared to a level of about 1 mmol/L in plasma; there is still too little phosphate in saliva to act as a significant buffer. The pH of unstimulated saliva is less than the pK_2 value of 7.2 for phosphate so that most of the phosphate is present as $H_2PO_4^-$ and cannot accept another hydrogen ion until the pH is close to 2.1, the pK_1 for phosphate.

2.6.3 Proteins

In saliva's plasma there is about one-thirtieth protein concentration as well as few amino acids with acidic or basic side chains which present an important buffering effect at the usual pH of the oral cavity.

2.6.4 pH

When the bicarbonate concentration increases, the salivary pH increases too. Henderson and Hasselbalch give the equation of the relationship between the pH and the bicarbonate concentration, which is $pH = pK + \log[HCO_3^-]/[H_2CO_3]$, in which the pK (about 6.1) and $[H_2CO_3]$ (about 1.2 mmol/L) are virtually independent of the flow rate. The latter is in equilibrium with the pCO_2 which, in saliva, is about the same as that in the venous blood. If we try to measure the pH of saliva, then it is very obligative to avoid exposure of the saliva to the atmosphere because the pH will be artificially elevated and CO_2 will be released. At very low flow rates, the pH of parotid saliva can be as low as 5.3, rising to 7.8 at very high flow rates. Because of the low bicarbonate concentration, patients with hyposalivation will have a low salivary buffering capacity and a low salivary pH (**Figure 3**).

2.6.5 Urea

The importance of salivary urea was acknowledged early in dental literature [35, 36]. The pH-raising effect of intraoral urea application was first described by Stefan [37]. This author found that in both in vivo and in vitro, urea could raise plaque pH up to pH 9 and that the addition of 40–50% urea to carbohydrates largely overcame the pH-lowering effect for up to 24 h. The value of salivary urea ranges from 2 to 6 mmol/L.

Urea possesses the capability to inhibit the metabolism and multiplication of bacteria in the saliva, which indirectly neutralize the acids in the oral environment and maintain the salivary acidobasic balance due to its buffer capacity [37, 38].

Less aciduric oral bacteria (*Streptococcus sanguinis* and *Streptococcus gordonii*) associated with dental health have the ability for alkali generation by hydrolyzing urea or arginine to **ammonia**. Production of ammonia is a mechanism that influences the balance remineralization-demineralization of the tooth, maintains neutral pH in oral cavity, and prevents the appearance of a cariogenic microflora [39, 40].

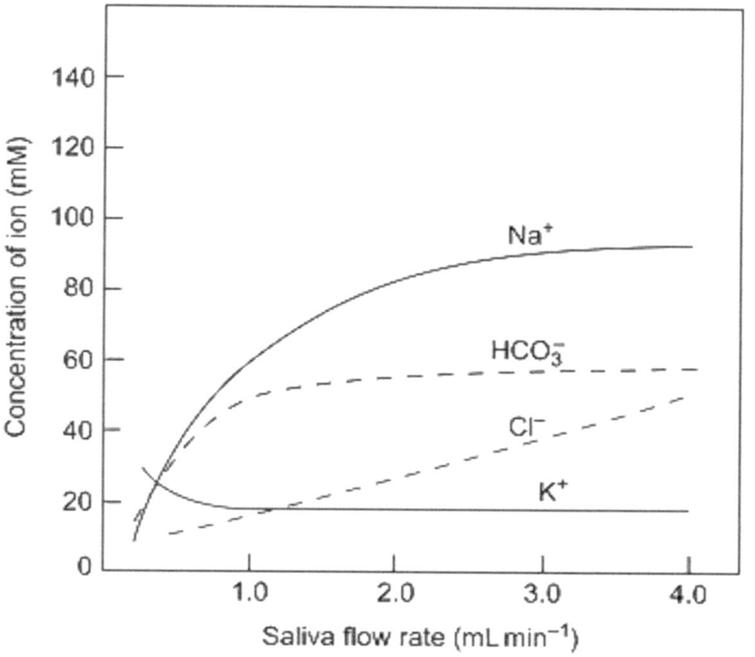

Figure 3.
The effects of flow rate on the concentrations of some components of saliva.

Urea can be used as a constituent of chewing gums for neutralized acids. Imfeld [41] explored the effect of sugar-free chewing gums containing various amounts of urea on the pH recovery in dental plaque.

After rinsing the mouth with 10 or 50% (w/v) sucrose solution, the respondents chewed the gum with different content of urea (10, 20, 30 mg) for 10 min. Increased value of salivary or plaque pH was found in the first minutes of chewing, and the effect of urea continued and lasted over 10 min. The higher concentrations of urea in chewing gum resulted in a faster leveling of the pH. As a result, the highest values of pH in the examined groups were observed in cases where they were treated with chewing gum containing 30 mg urea. With the use of such chewing gum, the salivary pH value does not fall below the level which is risky for the occurrence of dental caries, and there is a positive effect of chewing on the salivary flow that also affects neutralizing the acids in saliva or plaque [42, 43]. For the purpose of demonstrating the effect it can have on unstimulated saliva, a mathematical model of the influence of salivary urea on dental plaque was constructed. Data from study indicated that urea present in unstimulated saliva has a significant effect on plaque pH by elevating and counteracting the fall of plaque pH in the fasting state. The correlation of higher salivary urea concentrations and low salivary caries activity was registered in patients with chronic renal disease. These patients, who have elevated salivary urea concentration, have a reduced incidence of dental caries [44].

2.6.6 Calcium and phosphate concentrations

Saliva contains a supersaturated solution of calcium and phosphate, which neutralizes acids. Some epidemiological studies have revealed that humans with relatively high Ca and P in their plaque experience correspondingly lower caries. Higher Ca concentration of plaque is associated with low caries incidence.

The process of undersaturation of the saliva with respect to tooth mineral content is a result of decreasing total phosphate concentration at high flow rates which would be bad for the teeth.

However, if the flow rate increases, then the saliva's pH increases together with the bicarbonate concentration, and therefore high pH is altered. In the proportions of four different phosphate species (H_3PO_4, $H_2PO_4^-$, HPO_4^{2-}, and PO_4^{3}) together with the fall in total phosphate concentration, there is a fall in $H2PO_4^-$ and a slight increase in HPO_4^{2-} but a dramatic increase in PO_4^{3-}, all as a result high pH. It is the PO_4^{3-} that is an important ionic species with respect to the solubility of tooth mineral. So, although the total level of phosphate falls with increasing flow rate, the concentration of PO_4^{3-} actually increases as much as 40-fold when flow rate increases from the unstimulated level to high flow rates. The three components (Ca^{2+}, PO_4^{3-}, and OH^-) increase with salivary flow if taking into consideration the components of the ion product determining the solubility of tooth mineral in saliva. The saliva is more effective in reducing demineralization and promoting remineralization of the teeth if the flow rate is higher as well as the potential for calculus formation.

3. Conclusion

It can be concluded that tooth decay is a disease of great importance for general health. As a result, strategies to reduce the risk for dental caries are extremely important. The strategies may involve decreasing the growth or activity of bacteria especially *S. mutans*. To do so, people need to change their daily diet. Parents should advise children to avoid eating between meals, especially food containing carbohydrate.

Diet and oral microflora are connected to caries along with host factors such as salivary composition and flow.

Diet rich in fermentable carbohydrates is responsible for causing caries. Sucrose is one of the most cariogenic sugars, and glucose and fructose have also been shown to be less cariogenic. The cariogenic potential of carbohydrate-containing foods depends on their stickiness characteristics, frequency, and amount.

The saliva with its components plays an important role in maintaining oral, especially dental, health. Saliva is a natural factor that protects against demineralization. Apart from the activity of human saliva in diluting, clearing, neutralizing, and buffering acids, it also reduces demineralization and enhances the remineralization process.

Saliva performs its mechanical cleaning and protective functions though several physical and biochemical mechanisms. Saliva has buffer capacity which neutralizes acids in the mouth. The carbonic acid/bicarbonate system is the most important buffer in stimulated saliva.

The urea contributes to maintaining the acidobasic balance of saliva and thus affects the incidence of caries.

Author details

Efka Zabokova Bilbilova
Faculty of Dentistry, Department of Pediatric and Preventive Dentistry, "Ss. Cyril and Methodius" University, University Dental Clinic Center "St. Panteleimon", Skopje, Republic of North Macedonia

*Address all correspondence to: efka_zabokova@hotmail.com

References

[1] Arens U. Oral Health, Diet and Other Factors: Report of the British Nutrition foundation Task Force. Amsterdam, New York: Elsevier; 1998

[2] Moynihan P. The interrelation between diet and oral health. Proceedings of the Nutrition Society. 2005;**64**:571-580

[3] Jurgensen N, Petersen PE. Oral health and the impact of sociobehavioural factors in a cross sectional survey of 12-year old school children in Laos. BMC Oral Health. 2009;**9**:29. DOI: 10.1186/1472-6831-9-29

[4] Tinanoff N, Palmer CA. Dietary determinants of dental caries and dietary recommendations for pre school children. Journal of Public Health Dentistry. 2000;**60**(3):197-206

[5] Moynihan P, Petersen PE. Diet, nutrition and the prevention of dental diseases. Public Health Nutrition. 2004;**7**:201-226. DOI: 10.1079/PHN2003589

[6] Harris R. Biology of the children of Hopewood house, Bowral, Australia. 4. Observations on dental caries experience extending over five years (1957-61). Journal of Dental Research. 1963;**42**:1387-1399

[7] Sheiham A. Dental caries affects body weight, growth and quality of life in pre-school children. British Dental Journal. 2006;**201**:625-626. DOI: 10.1038/sj.bdj.4814259

[8] Gustafsson B, Quensel C, Lanke L. The Vipeholm dental caries study: The effect of different levels of carbohydrate intake on caries activity in 436 individuals observed for five years. Acta Odontologica Scandinavica. 1954;**11**(3-4):232-264

[9] Linke HA, Birchmeier RI. Effect of increasing sucrose concentrations on oral lactic acid production. Annals of Nutrition & Metabolism. 2000;**44**:121-124

[10] Bernabé E, Vehkalahti MM, Sheiham A, Lundqvist A, Suominen AL. The shape of the dose-response relationship between sugars and caries in adults. Journal of Dental Research. 2016;**95**:167-172

[11] Marshall T, Levy S, Broffitt B, et al. Dental caries and beverage consumption in young children. Pediatric Dental Journal. 2003;**112**(3):184-191

[12] Mobley C, Marshall TA, Milgrom P, Coldwell SE. The contribution of dietary factors to dental caries and disparities in caries. Academic Pediatrics. 2009;**9**(6):410-414. DOI: 10.1016/j.acap.2009.09.008

[13] Decker RT, Loveren CV. Sugars and dental caries. The American Journal of Clinical Nutrition. 2003;**78**(Suppl):881S-892S

[14] Burt B, Eklund S, Morgan K. The effects of sugars intake and frequency of ingestion on dental caries increment in a three-year longitudinal study. Journal of Dental Research. 1988;**67**(11):1422-1429

[15] Lingström P, van Houte J, Kashket S. Food starches and dental caries. Critical Reviews in Oral Biology and Medicine. 2000;**11**(3):366-380

[16] Shils ME, Shike M, Ross AC, et al. Modern Nutrition in Health and Disease. 10th ed. Philadelphia, PA: Lippincott, Williams & Wilkins; 2006

[17] Dodds MWJ, Edgar WM. Effects of dietary sucrose levels on pH fall and acid-ion profile in human dental plaque after a starch mouth-rinse. Archives of Oral Biology. 1986;**31**:509-512

[18] Rugg-Gunn AJ. Diet and dental caries. In: Murray JJ, editor. Prevention

of Oral Disease. Oxford: Oxford University Press; 1996. pp. 3-3146

[19] Dennison BA. Fruit juice consumption by infants and children: A review. Journal of the American College of Nutrition. 1996;**15**(5):26-29

[20] Sohn W, Burt B, Sowers M. Carbonated soft drinks and dental caries in the primary dentition. Journal of Dental Research. 2006;**85**(3):262-266

[21] Kolker J, Yuan Y, Burt B, et al. Dental caries and dietary patterns in low-income African American children. Pediatric Dental Journal. 2007;**29**(6):457-464

[22] Marshall TA, Eichenberger-Gilmore JM, Broffitt B, Warren JJ, Levy SM. Dental caries and childhood obesity: Roles of diet and socio-economic status. Community Dentistry and Oral Epidemiology. 2007;**35**:449-458

[23] Kleinberg I. Oral effects of sugars and sweeteners. International Dental Journal. 1985;**35**:180-189

[24] Kashket S, Zhang J, van Houte J. Accumulation of fermentable sugars and metabolic acids in food particles that become entrapped on the dentition. Journal of Dental Research. 1996;**75**:1885-1891

[25] Palmer C, Kent R, Loo C, et al. Diet and caries-associated bacteria in severe early childhood caries. Journal of Dental Research. 2010;**89**(11):1224-1229

[26] Murray J, Rugg-Gunn A, Jenkins G. Fluorides in Caries Prevention. 3rd ed. Oxford, UK: Butterworth-Heinemann; 1991

[27] Carmichael CL, French AD, Rugg-Gunn A, Furness JA. The relationship between social class and caries experience in five-year-old children in Newcastle and Northumberland after twelve years of fluoridation. Community Dental Health. 1984;**1**:47-54

[28] van Loveren C. Sugar restriction for caries prevention: Amount and frequency. Which is more important? Caries Research. 2019;**53**:168-175. DOI: 10.1159/000489571

[29] Moynihan P, Makino Y, Petersen PE, Ogawa H. Implications of WHO guideline on sugars for dental health professionals. Community Dentistry and Oral Epidemiology. 2018;**46**:1-7

[30] Leone WC, Oppenheim GF. Physical and chemical aspects of saliva as indicators of risk for dental caries in humans. Journal of Dental Education. 2001;**65**(10):1054-1062

[31] Dawes C, Dong C. The flow rate and electrolyte composition of whole saliva elicited by the use of sucrose-containing and sugar-free chewing-gums. Archives of Oral Biology. 1995;**40**:699-705

[32] Tanzer J, Grant L, McMahon T. Bicarbonate-based dental powder, fluoride and saccharin inhibition of dental caries associated with S. mutans infection of rats. Journal of Dental Research. 1988;**67**:969-972

[33] Bardow A, Moe D, Nyvad B, Nauntofte B. The buffer capacity and buffer systems of human whole saliva measured without loss of CO2. Archives of Oral Biology. 2000;**45**:1-12

[34] Bardow A, Hofer E, Nyvad B, Cate JM, Kirkeby S, Moe D, et al. Effect of saliva composition on experimental root caries. Caries Research. 2005;**39**:71-77

[35] Nauntofte B, Tenovuo JO, Lagerlöf F. Secretion and composition of saliva. In: Fejerskov O, EAM K, editors. Dental Caries The Disease and its Clinical Management. Oxford: Blackwell, Munksgaard; 2003. pp. 7-27

[36] Arends J, Jongebloed WL, Goldberg M, Schuthof J. Interaction of urea and human enamel. Caries Research. 1984;**18**:17-24

[37] Macpherson LMD, Dawes C. Urea concentration in minor mucous gland secretions and the effect of salivary film velocity on urea metabolism by streptococcus vestibularis in an artificial plaque. Journal of Periodontal Research. 1991;**26**:395-401

[38] Sjögren K, Ruben J, Lingstrom P, Lundberg AB, Birkhed D. Fluoride and urea chewing gums in an intra-oral experimental caries model. Caries Research. 2002;**36**:64-69

[39] Dawes C, Dibdin GH. Salivary concentrations of urea released from a chewing gum containing urea and how these affect the urea content of gel-stabilized plaques and their pH after exposure to sucrose. Caries Research. 2001;**35**:344-353

[40] Leone CW, Oppenheim FG. Physical and chemical aspects of saliva as indicators of risk for dental caries in human. Journal of Dental Education. 2001;**65**:1054-1064

[41] Imfeld T, Birkhed D, Lingstrom P. Effect of urea in sugar – Free chewing gums on pH recovery in human dental plaque evaluated with three different methods. Caries Research. 1995;**29**:172-180

[42] Raymond G, Schipper A, Erika Silletti A, Vingerhoeds MH. Saliva as research material: Biochemical, physiochemical, and practical aspects. Archives of Oral Biology. 2007;**52**:1114-1135

[43] Zabokova-Bibilova E, Sotirovska-Ivkovska A, Ambarkova V. Correlation between salivary urea level and dental caries. Contributions. 2012;**33**(1):289-302

[44] Dibdin GH, Dawes C. A mathematical model of the influence of salivary urea on the pH of fasted dental plaque and on the changes occurring during a cariogenic challenge. Caries Research. 1998;**32**:70-74

Chapter 3

Characterization and Virulence of *Candida* Isolated from Children with Dental Caries and Its Susceptibility to Various Antimicrobial Agents

M.S. Beena

Abstract

Candida is known to be associated with early colonization of cariogenic microorganisms leading to dental caries and there is a need to determine the effectiveness of various chemotherapeutic agents against it. The study is aimed to isolate, characterize *Candida* from the dental plaque of children with dental caries, to study its virulence factors and the antimicrobial activity of coconut oil, probiotics, 0.2% chlorhexidine and ketoconazole on *C. albicans*. Samples were collected using sterile cotton swabs from children with dental caries and streaked on Sabouraud's dextrose agar plates and incubated at 37°C for 24 h. Candidal colonies were isolated, species identified, and virulence factors tested, and its susceptibility to 0.2% chlorhexidine, probiotics, coconut oil, and ketoconazole was determined using disc diffusion method. *C. albicans* was the predominant species isolated, and virulence factors such as phospholipase, hemolysin, germ tube, and hyphal formation were seen. The mean zone of inhibition for chlorhexidine was found to be 21.8 mm, for coconut oil it was 16.8 mm, for probiotics it was 13.5 mm, and for ketoconazole it was 22.3 mm. The difference between the groups was not statistically significant. Thus chlorhexidine and coconut oil were found to exhibit significant antimicrobial activity which is comparable with ketoconazole.

Keywords: *Candida albicans*, virulence, children with dental caries, antifungal susceptibility, hemolysis, phospholipase

1. Introduction

Dental caries is defined as an infectious microbiological disease of the teeth that results in localized dissolution and destruction of the calcified tissue [1]. Dental plaque (biofilm) is defined as a soft thin film of food debris, mucin, and epithelial cells that adheres to the tooth surface, providing the medium for the growth of various bacterial species [1]. The term "cariogenic bacteria" refers to certain pathogenic microorganisms, which have the ability to ferment the carbohydrates and produce acids as a by-product [1]. Microflora responsible for caries development usually belongs to the normal physiologic flora with a low cariogenic potential (low virulence). But changes in the oral environment leading to a shift in the balance between the cariogenic microflora, host defenses such as resistance and acid susceptibility of the tooth, plaque and saliva increase the cariogenic potential of the microflora (increase its virulence) and initiate caries.

Streptococcus mutans have been implicated as the most important bacteria for caries initiation and its progression. They exhibit a number of virulent characteristics that makes the plaque or biofilm cariogenic. They produce various acids, especially lactic acid, which demineralizes the tooth enamel. They also produce extracellular polysaccharides that allow for further plaque growth. In addition to S. *mutans*, *Lactobacilli* and the yeasts are important in the pathogenesis of dental caries.

Candida is a normal commensal in the oral cavity and participates in the formation of complex microbial oral biofilm. The percentage of *Candida* species colonization ranges from 20 to 40% in healthy individuals to about 60% in immuno-compromised people where it becomes the predominant flora [2]. Poor oral hygiene, increase in the intake of sugary foods and presence of carious lesions in children, favors candidal colonization [3]. The microbiology of dental plaque resulting in dental caries has been researched extensively. *Candida* seems to play an important role in microbial adherence to dental surfaces in coaggregation with *S. mutans* [4]. The synergistic action of *Candida* along with mutans streptococci enhances its cariogenicity and its adherence to the oral biofilm and carious tooth substance [4–7]. *C. albicans* is found to ferment glucose and maltose, producing both acid and gas and its contribution to overall microbial acid production seems to be important . Other factors attributing to the cariogenic ability of Candida are its adherence to saliva proteins, ability to penetrate into dentinal canals, and its enzymatic activity to degrade collagen [5]. *C. albicans* is known to be associated with dental caries, but more recently the role of nonalbicans candida (NAC) including *C. glabrata, C. guilliermondii*, *C. krusei*, C. *kyfer*, and *C. tropicalis* in the development of dental caries has been reported [3–9].

Research on the chemotherapeutic approaches to reduce the levels of *C. albicans* resulting in dental caries has been limited, and there is a need to determine the effectiveness of various chemotherapeutic agents against it. Ketoconazole is an antifungal imidazole compound which has been found to be very active against both superficial and systemic fungal infections. The inhibitory effect of ketoconazole on *C. albicans*, as determined by incomplete respiration or impairment of respiratory function, occurred at the lowest concentration observed among the imidazole compounds [10]. So it is taken as a standard drug against which others are compared.

Chlorhexidine is a biocide that is widely prescribed in dentistry both as an antiseptic mouthwash and a denture disinfectant. It has a broad spectrum of antimicrobial activity against a variety of organisms, including *C. albicans*. It acts as a fungicide leading to the coagulation of nucleoproteins and changes in cell walls allowing the escape of cytoplasmic components through the plasmalemma. It is also capable of inhibiting candidal adhesion to biological and inert surfaces [11]. Coconut (*Cocos nucifera*), the unique source of various natural products is consumed as a part of the staple diet in many countries and useful for the development of medicines against various diseases. The parts of its fruit like coconut kernel and tender coconut water are of a great medicinal value because of its antimicrobial and antioxidant property [12]. Lauric acid, a medium chain fatty acid (MCF), which is predominant in coconut oil, has proved to have antimicrobial, antiviral, and anti-inflammatory action. Probiotics can be defined as living microbes, or as food ingredients containing living microbes, that beneficially influence the health of the host when used in adequate numbers [13]. They have been used to modify microfloral ecosystems and have shown some success as a therapeutic for oral diseases.

The study aims to isolate, characterize *Candida* from the dental plaque attached to the tooth surfaces of children with dental caries, to study its virulence factors, and to test the susceptibility of *C. albicans* to ketoconazole, 0.2% chlorhexidine, probiotics, and coconut oil, and to compare their antimicrobial efficacy.

2. Materials and methods

Subjects for the study were selected from the children who consulted the out-patient Department of Pediatric and Preventive Dentistry, Kannur Dental College, Anjarakandy. Based on the caries experience (dmfs index) that was recorded using visible light, mouth mirror, and CPI probe, 50 children with dental caries were selected for the study. Informed written consent was obtained from the parent/guardian of the children. Exclusion criteria included the children who were on topical or systemic antibiotics or antifungal medication. This study was reviewed and approved by the Institutional Ethical Committee of Kannur Medical College.

2.1 Armamentarium

1. Mouth mirror
2. Explorer, Tweezer
3. Sterile Cotton swabs
4. Magnifying glass
5. Culture media-Sabouraud's Dextrose Agar, Corn Meal Agar, Hichrome Agar (HI MEDIA), Mueller Hinton Agar, Blood Agar
6. Serum
7. Culture plates
8. Stock vials
9. Glass slide
10. Cover slips
11. Incubator
12. Light microscope
13. Saline solution
14. Filter paper discs
15. 2% ketoconazole (KevonR)
16. 0.2% chlorhexidine (Hexidine mouthwash)
17. Probiotics (VizylacR, lactic acid *Bacillus* 120×10^6)
18. Coconut oil

Samples were collected using sterile cotton swabs. Swabbing was done over the buccal, lingual, proximal, and cervical portion of the tooth and immediately transferred to the lab for microbiological analysis. The samples were inoculated for culture on Sabouraud's Dextrose Agar (SDA) plates supplemented with 1% chloramphenicol with pH 6.6 to prevent bacterial overgrowth. The plates were incubated at 37°C for 24–72 h. Isolates were identified by colony morphology on SDA plates. Growth appears in 1 to 2 days as creamy, smooth, convex pasty colonies with a moldy odor. Culture is said to be negative if there is no growth even after 72 h of incubation. The positive cultures were stocked in SDA stock vials (**Figure 1**).

Isolates were speciated based on the conventional methods of germ tube test and Corn Meal Agar (Dalmau Plate Culture Technique) and by Hichrom Agar-Candida Differential Media. For germ tube test, a small portion of an isolated colony of the yeast to be tested was inoculated into the 0.5 ml human serum and incubated at

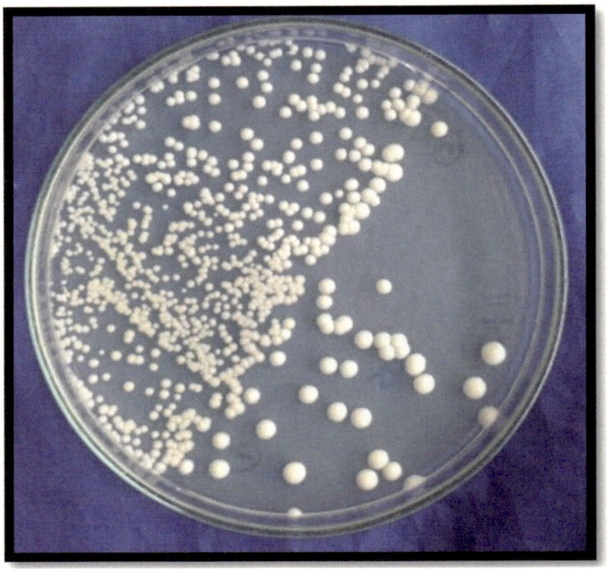

Figure 1.
Growth of Candida *on SDA.*

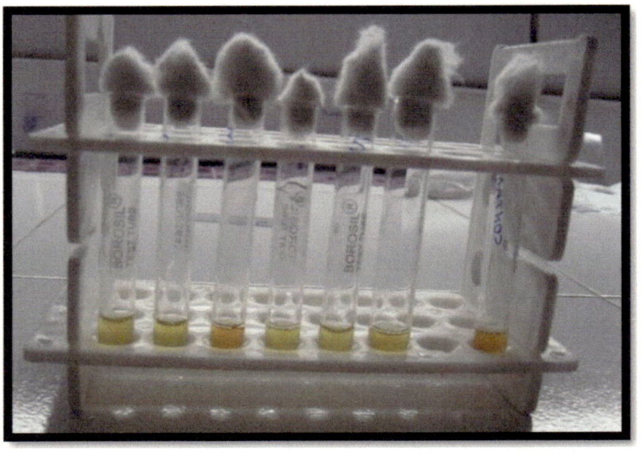

Figure 2.
Inoculation of Candida *in human serum for germ tube testing.*

DOI: http://dx.doi.org/10.5772/intechopen.91912

37°C for 2 h (**Figure 2**). After 2 h of incubation, a drop of the yeast serum suspension was placed on a glass slide, overlaid with a cover slip and examined microscopically for the presence of germ tube under low power microscope. Test is said to be positive if tube like extensions from the yeast cell is seen within 2 h of inoculation and the isolate was considered as *C. albicans.* For Corn Meal Agar (Dalmau Plate Culture Technique), an isolated colony from the primary culture media was picked using a straight wire and inoculated into cornmeal agar plate at 45° angles to the culture media. A sterile cover slip was placed over the surface of the agar, covering a portion of the inoculated streaks (**Figure 3**).

The plates were incubated at 28°C for 48 h. The areas where the agar was streaked were examined under microscope. Isolates with large, highly refractile thick walled cell, single or multiple, terminal or intercalary chlamydospores were identified as *C. albicans* (**Figure 4**). Species identification was also done by streaking the samples on HiCrome Agar media (Himedia, India) and incubated at 37°C for 24 h. Colonies were identified depending on their color and pattern of growth.

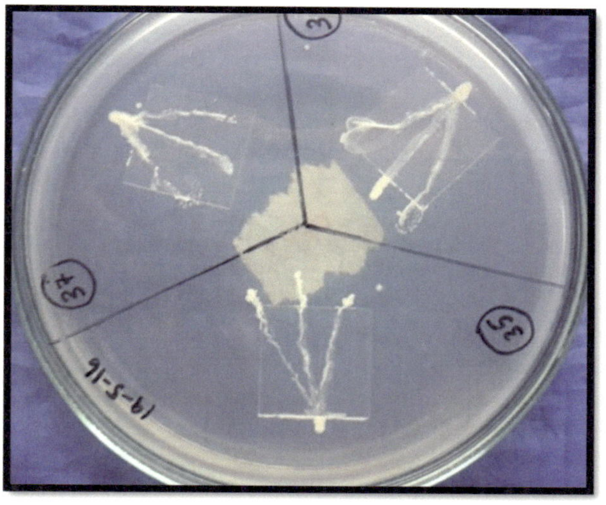

Figure 3.
Dalmau plate culture on Corn Meal Agar.

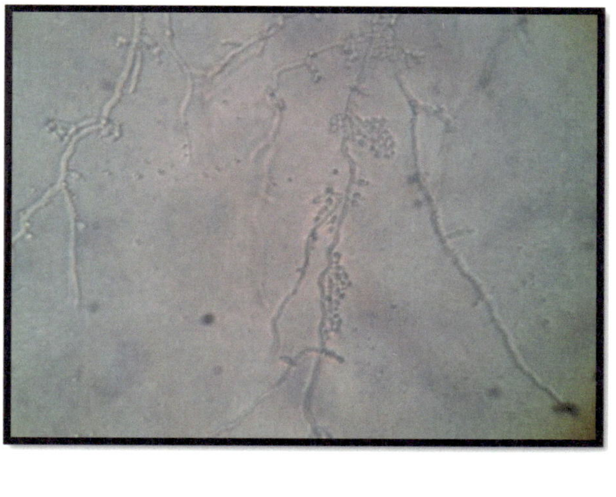

Figure 4.
Chlamydospore formation of C. albicans*-microscopic view (high power).*

The virulence markers like hemolysis and phospholipase were tested on the *Candidal* isolates. For hemolysis test, the Candidal isolates were seeded onto blood agar enriched with 1% glucose and incubated at 37°C for 48 h in a 5% CO_2 atmosphere. Hemolytic activity was defined as the formation of a translucent halo around the colonies. To determine phospholipase activity, test medium containing 65 g SDA, 58.4 g NaCl, and 5.5 g $CaCl_2$ was dissolved in 980 ml distilled water and sterilized at 121°C for 12 min [9]. Egg yolk was centrifuged at 5000*g* for 30 min. The supernatant was removed and added to cooled medium (45–50°C) (2%), mixed, and dispensed in plates. An aliquot (10 μl) of the yeasts suspension was inoculated onto test medium and incubated at 37°C for 4 days. Colony diameter and colony diameter plus precipitation zone were measured for each isolate and the zone of phospholipase activity was calculated [14] (**Figure 5**).

$$\text{Pz} = \frac{\text{Colony diameter}}{\text{Colony diameter} + \text{Zone of Precipitation}} \tag{1}$$

Five classes were described for phospholipase activity including;
Pz value = 1 means that the test strain is negative for phospholipase,
Pz <0.90–0.99 = weak phospholipase activity (+),
Pz = 0.80–0.89 = poor phospholipase activity (++);
Pz = 0.70–0.79 = moderate phospholipase activity (+++) and
Pz < 0.70 = large phospholipase activity (++++).

Kirby Bauer's Disc Diffusion method is used to test the antifungal activity of 2% ketoconazole (KevonR), 0.2% chlorhexidine (Hexidine mouthwash), probiotics (VizylacR, lactic acid *Bacillus* 120 × 10^6), and coconut oil against *C. albicans.* Suspensions of *C. albicans* were prepared in saline solution adjusted to the turbidity of 0.5 McFarland and streaked onto Mueller-Hinton agar supplemented with 1% glucose evenly. 0.2% chlorhexidine, coconut oil and probiotics (Vizylac, lactic acid *Bacillus*), and 2% ketoconazole were applied on filter paper discs of 6 mm separately (4.0 μL/disc) and allowed to dry. Then the discs of chlorhexidine, coconut oil, probiotics, and ketoconazole are placed on its surface at equal distance and

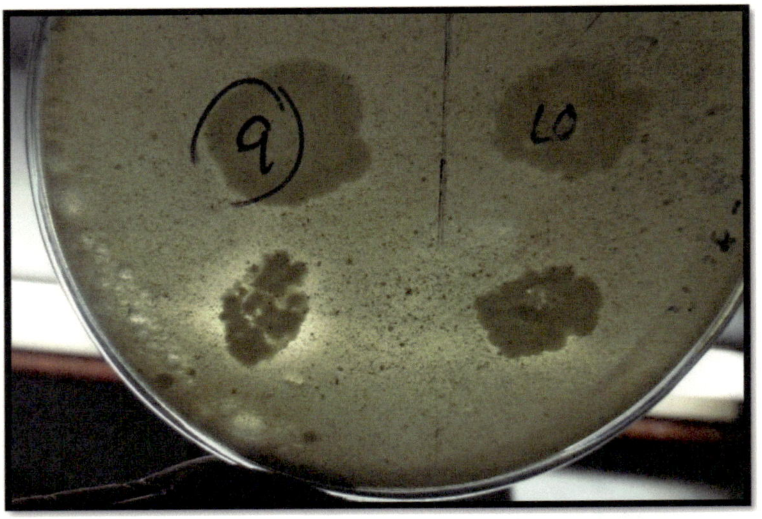

Figure 5.
Phospholipase test.

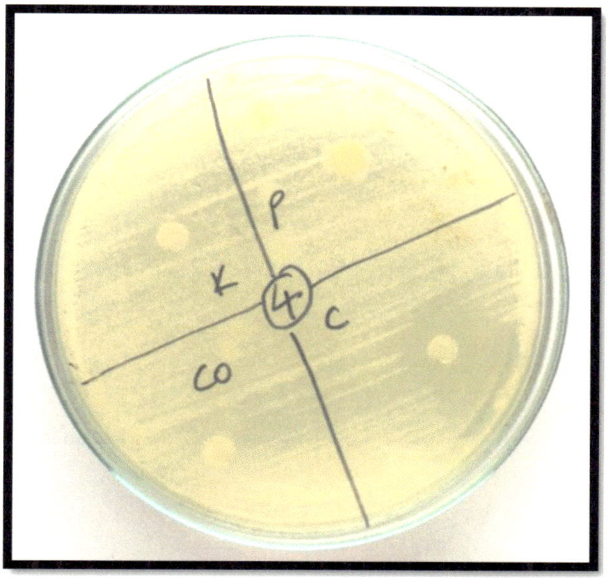

Figure 6.
Zone of inhibition observed around the discs.

incubated at 37°C for 24 h. Twenty isolates of *C. albicans* were tested in this manner. The zone of inhibition around the discs was observed (**Figure 6**), which will be measured and compared.

The phenotypes and the susceptibility of the isolates to the antifungals were compared against one another by the nonparametric Kruskal-Wallis, for multiple independent groups, or Mann-Whitney, for two independent groups, tests. The results were considered statistically significant at $P \leq 0.05$.

3. Results

Candida was identified by its morphological features of cream, smooth, pasty convex colonies with a moldy odor on SDA. Candidal carriage among the children was found to be 84% (42 children-positive), and *C. albicans* was found to be the predominant species identified. The presence of *C. albicans* was confirmed by observing the Germ tube formation and the formation of chlamydospore. On HiCrome agar, *C. albicans* were seen as light green-colored smooth colonies, *C. tropicalis* as metallic blue-colored raised colonies, *C. glabrata* as cream smooth colonies, and *C. krusei* appeared as purple fuzzy colonies (**Figure 7**). The distribution of various species of *Candida* identified is given in **Table 1** and **Figure 8**.

Virulence factors such as hemolysin, phospholipase, and germ tube formation were expressed by the *Candidal* isolates in the study. Phospholipase was tested positive in 92.8% of the isolates, hemolysis in 4.76%, and germ tube and hyphal formation in 5.76% as seen in **Table 2** and **Figure 9**. When various species were analyzed for their virulence factors, it was seen that 8% *C. albicans* showed hemolysis, 96% of them were positive for phospholipase test and all of them showed germ tube and hyphal formation. Hemolysis and germ tube formation was not detected in the rest of the species of Candida. For phospholipase, all the isolates of *C. tropicalis*, C. *guilliermondii*, *C. glabrata*, and C. *kyfer* and 60% of isolates of *C. krusei* showed phospholipase production (**Table 3**).

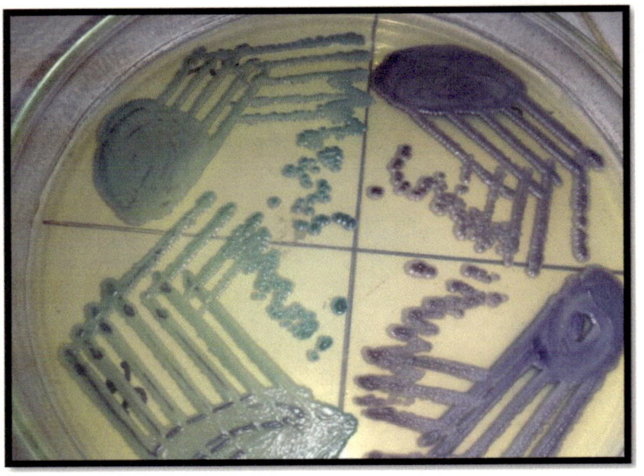

Figure 7.
Candidal colonies on HiChrome Agar.

Species	Frequency (%)
Candida albicans	25 (59.5)
Candida glabrata	3 (7.1)
Candida guilliermondii	1 (2.4)
Candida krusei	5 (11.9)
Candida kyfer	1 (2.4)
Candida tropicalis	7 (16.7)
Total	42(100)

Table 1.
Comparison of species distribution of Candida *among the children with dental caries.*

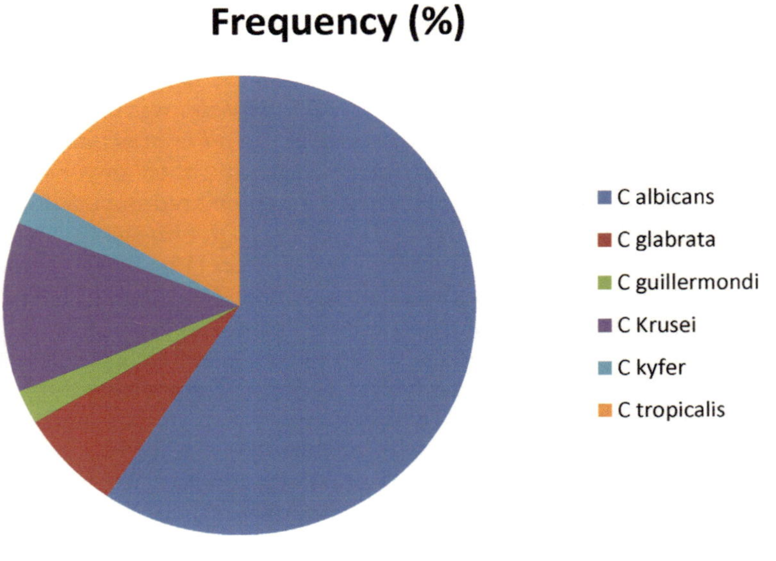

Figure 8.
Species distribution of Candida.

Virulence factors	Number (%)
Phospholipase test	
Positive	39 (92.8)
Negative	3 (7.14)
Hemolysis test	
Positive	2 (4.76)
Negative	40 (95.2)
Germ tube and hyphal formation	
Positive	25(59.52)
Negative	17 (40.47)

Table 2.
Virulence factors exhibited by Candida *isolates.*

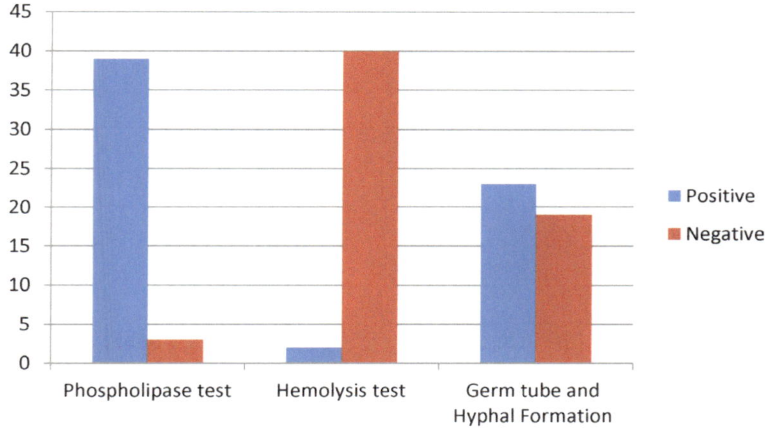

Figure 9.
Virulence factors of Candida.

Species of Candida	N	Hemolysis test		Phospholipase		Germtube and hyphal formation	
		P(%)	N(%)	P(%)	N(%)	P(%)	N(%)
C. albicans	25	2(8)	23(92)	24(96)	1(4)	25(100)	0 (0)
C. tropicalis	7	0 (0)	7(100)	7(100)	0 (0)	0 (0)	7(100)
C. guilliermondii	1	0 (0)	1(100)	1(100)	0 (0)	0 (0)	1(100)
C. krusei	5	0 (0)	5(100)	3(60)	2(40)	0 (0)	5(100)
C. glabrata	3	0 (0)	3(100)	3(100)	0 (0)	0 (0)	3(100)
C. kyfer	1	0 (0)	1(100)	1(100)	0 (0)	0 (0)	1(100)
Total	42	2(4.76)	40(95.2)	39 (92.8)	3(7.14)	25 (59.52)	19(40.47)

Table 3.
Virulence factors exhibited by individual species of Candida P-Positive , N-Negative.

The antifungal susceptibility test showed that *C. albicans* was susceptible to ketoconazole, chlorhexidine, coconut oil, and probiotics by having a clear zone of inhibition. **Table 4** shows comparison of zone of inhibition between different

Antimicrobial agents	N	Mean (mm)	Std. deviation	Chi-square	P value
Ketoconazole	20	22.30	15.076	7.429	0.059NS
Chlorhexidine	20	21.80	8.458		
Coconut oil	20	16.80	12.846		
Probiotics	20	13.50	13.656		
Total	80	18.60	13.033		

Table 4.
Comparison of zone of inhibition of antimicrobial agents against Candida albicans *NS: not significant Kruskal-Walla ANOVA.*

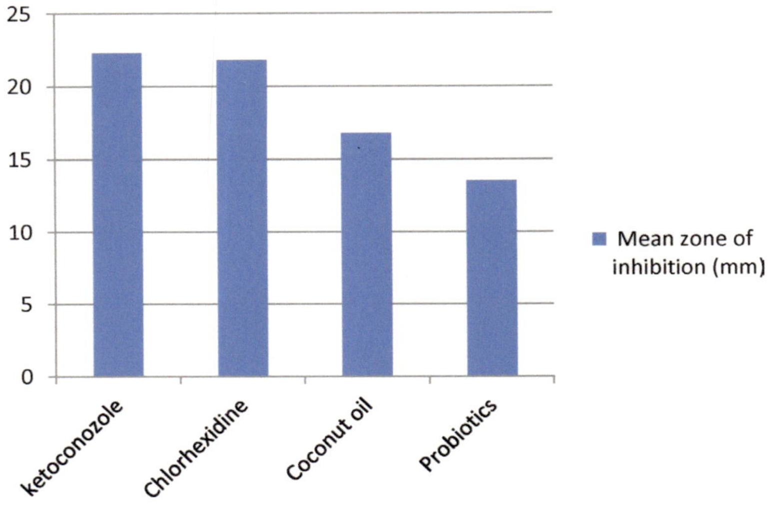

Figure 10.
Mean zone of inhibition of the antimicrobial agents against Candida albicans.

Antimicrobial agents	N	Mean	Std. deviation	Mean difference	Z-value	P value*
Ketoconazole	20	22.30	15.076	−0.5	−0.611	0.542
Chlorhexidine	20	21.80	8.458			
**Mann-Whitney U test.*						

Table 5.
Comparison of zone of inhibition between ketoconazole and chlorhexidine.

Antimicrobial agents	N	Mean	Std. deviation	Mean difference	Z-value	P value*
Ketoconazole	20	22.30	15.076	−5.5	−1.761	0.078
Coconut oil	20	16.80	12.846			
**Mann-Whitney U test.*						

Table 6.
Comparison of zone of inhibition between ketoconazole and coconut oil.

Antimicrobial agents	N	Mean	Std. deviation	Mean difference	Z-value	P value*
Ketoconazole	20	22.30	15.076	−8.8	−2.272	0.023
Probiotics	20	13.50	13.656			

**Mann-Whitney U test.*

Table 7.
Comparison of zone of inhibition between ketoconazole and probiotics.

groups. It was found that the mean zone of inhibition for ketoconazole was 22.3 mm, while it was 21.8 mm for chlorhexidine, 16.8 mm for coconut oil, and 13.5 mm for probiotics (**Figure 10**). The difference between the groups was not statistically significant (Chi-square value 7.42, *P* value 0.06).

The comparison of the zone of inhibition between ketoconazole and chlorhexidine showed that the mean zone of inhibition for ketoconazole was 22.3 mm, whereas for chlorhexidine, it was 21.8 mm. The difference was not statistically significant (*P* value 0.54) (**Table 5**). The comparison of the zone of inhibition between ketoconazole and coconut oil also showed no statistically significant difference (*P* value 0.07) (**Table 6**). However, in the comparison of the zone of inhibition of ketoconazole and probiotics, there was found to be a statistically significant difference between the groups (*P* value 0.02) (**Table 7**).

4. Discussion

Candida species colonizes the oral cavity of infants. Transmissions by mother during childbirth, pacifier use, and feeding habits are factors related to *Candida* oral colonization [15]. A study by Xiao revealed that mothers of the children affected by Early Childhood Caries (ECC) also have high *C. albicans* carriage, and most of the children were carrying the same *C. albicans* strains as their mothers [16].

The age of infection plays an important role in the disease process and the optimal period to intervene with preventive strategies [17].

Candida is a common commensal of the normal oral microbiota [18]. It is an opportunistic pathogen and has the ability to cause a variety of infections in immuno-compromised hosts like oral candidiasis which manifests as oral thrush in infants and chronic atrophic candidiasis in adults. Its ability to exist both in yeast and pseudohyphal/hyphal form plays an important role in its virulence [19]. While yeast form is a normal commensal of the oral cavity, pseudohyphal (budding shape) is associated with a fungal (saprophytic) condition, and the presence of hyphal forms is seen to be associated with active symptomatic infections. It displays many pathogenic forms due to which it is capable of adhering to various surfaces of host organisms, interfering with their immunological system, and producing several catabolytes [20].

Candida spp. is acidogenic and has the ability to ferment carbohydrates. Klinke et al. [4] have shown that in an environment with a pH below 5.5, which is relevant for ECC formation, acidification by *S. mutans* decreases considerably and ceases around pH 4.2, whereas *Candida* can still secrete acid at pH 4.0. It also produces several organic acids including pyruvic acid and acetate [21]. Abundant H + ATPase on the plasma membrane of yeasts pumping out proteins from the cell is induced by glucose and makes a contribution to the acidification [22]. Furthermore, it was shown that *Candida* was capable of dissolving the hydroxyapatite at an approximately 20-fold rate higher than *S. mutans*, despite a lower number of yeast cells in the culture [4, 5, 7–20]. Acidification causing demineralization of dental tissues plays a major role in the progression of dental caries. The potential of *C. albicans* to adhere to saliva proteins and *S. mutans*, its acid producing capability, its ability to penetrate into dentinal canals, and its enzymatic activity to degrade collagen indicates its cariogenic ability and possible role in the progression of dental caries.

Of the different species of *Candida*, the most prevalent one recovered from the oral cavity is *C. albicans.* Identification of infecting strains of *Candida* is important because isolates of *Candida* species differ widely in their ability to cause infection as well as in their susceptibility to antifungal agents [23]. Hence, the present study is undertaken to identify and to characterize *Candida* species, to study its virulence factors and the antimicrobial activity of coconut oil, probiotics, 0.2% chlorhexidine, and ketoconazole on *C. albicans*.

Candidal growth was observed to be 84% among the ECC children, whereas it was only 24% among the caries free group. The results show that there is significant association between the Candidal carriage and the presence of ECC. This is in correlation with the previous studies by Hossain et al. [24], de Carvalho [20], Tony Jose [25], Ann Thomas [26], Fragkou et al. [5], and others. However in the studies by Maijala et al. [27], Peretz et al. [28], and Ratson et al. [29], no significant association between *Candida* and dental caries was found. This could be attributed to factors like difference in saliva rate, composition, buffering capacity etc. that influence the carious process. And it was observed that these authors employed other technical methods for detection of yeasts in the carious tooth samples and did not make cultures to identify them, which is considered to be a gold standard method for detection of yeast. But in the present study, a correlation between the caries experience of the children and *Candida* in terms of isolation frequency and numbers was observed, this being in line with most previous findings. And based on the fact that *Candida* is able to colonize the tooth surface, invade the dentinal tubules [30], produce a large amount of acids provoking demineralization of the dental enamel [21], and dissolution of hydroxyapatite [7], it has been hypothesized that *C. albicans* is a relevant pathogen involved in the progression of caries [27]. *C. albicans* also actively participates in cariogenic biofilms, through synergistic interaction with S. *mutans.* Evidence of enhanced exopolymeric matrix production, facilitated by the increased surface area associated with hyphal networks, supports mixed biofilm growth of dense communities cemented to tooth enamel, thus causing progression of dental caries [31].

The Candidal carriage in the present study (84%) is lesser than that of studies conducted by Merchant et al. [5] and Ann Thomas [26], where the prevalence of *Candida* species in ECC children was found to be 89 and 100% respectively. It was observed that the present study showed higher rate of Candidal carriage when compared to the studies by Hodson and Craig [32], Hossain et al. [24], de Carvalho [20], and Tony Jose [25], where the *Candida* carriage in ECC was found to be in the range of 56–67%. The differences in living environment, ecological environment of the oral cavity, and geographical variation and food habits of individuals might have influenced this variation among the rate of Candidal carriage among different studies [20].

The *Candida* species growth among the caries free children was observed to be 24% in this study. This is in correlation with the previous studies by Merchant et al. [5], Rozkiewicz [33], Jose [25], Thomas [26], Hossain [24], where the *Candida* frequency among those without caries was found to be in the range of 2–38%. The frequency of yeast carriage also varies due to differences in age, body fluids, mucosal surface, and natural barriers against yeast colonization [20].

5. Distribution of candida species

Even though *C. albicans* is recognized as the most prevalent species, many other species of *Candida* are identified with a potential clinical importance as they differ in the expression of virulence factors and antifungal susceptibility. Non *albicans Candida* species (NAC) are on the rise due to increasing immuno-compromised states [34]. Different species of *Candida* differ in their adherence to the oral tissues and hence their virulence.

Both conventional methods like germ tube test and chlamydospore formation on Dalmau plate culture and more advanced methods like CHROM AGAR *Candida* differential media (Hi Media) were used in the present study, for differentiation between different species of *Candida*. *C. albicans* was identified by the formation of germ tube and chlamydospores. CHROM AGAR is a relatively rapid method to differentiate between different *Candida* species. It facilitates the detection and identification of *Candida* species from mixed culture and provides result in 24–48 h. Previous studies shows that the sensitivity and specificity of CHROM agar for *Candida albicans* were 100 and 96%, *C. tropicalis* were 100 and 100%, *C. krusei* were 100 and 100%, and *C. glabrata* 75 and 100%, respectively [34].

The overall distribution of *Candida* species among the isolates was observed as follows: *C. albicans* (61.1%), *C. glabrata* (5.6%), C. *guilliermondii* (3.7%), *C. krusei* (11.1%), C. *kyfer* (3.7%), and *C. tropicalis* (14.8%). No isolates of *C. dubliniensis* was observed in the present study, which is similar to the studies by Moreira et al. [35], Martins et al. [36], de Carvalho [20], Al Hebshi et al. [37, 38], and Cortelli et al. [39]. But in the studies by Jabra Rizk et al. [40], Al Ahmed et al. [41], and Moraga et al. [42], C. *dubliniensis* was found in statistically significant proportions in caries active children. C. *dubliniensis* that shares a similar morphology with *C. albicans* is not frequently detected in various studies due to difficulty in differentiating between these yeast species, and it is more commonly isolated from immuno-compromised – HIV positive subjects [43]. However Kniest et al. [38] reported a case of isolating C. *dubliniensis* from plaque and carious dentine of a healthy 5 year old boy.

In the present study, *C. tropicalis* was found to be the most predominant among the Non *albicans Candida* species (14.8%), which is in correlation with the studies by de Carvalho [20], Cortelli et al. [39], Martins et al. [36], and Al Hebshi et al. [37]. However in the study by Al Hebshi et al. [38], *C. krusei* was most prevalent (6.9%) with the lowest counts for *C. tropicalis* (3.1%), and in a study done by Jabra Rizk et al. [40], *C. glabrata* (23%) was predominant. *C. kusei* is found in significant proportions in HIV and leprosy patients, and it is intrinsically resistant to the widely used triazole antifungal fluconazole and poses therapeutic problems [44]. An extensive diversity in the nonalbicans species was observed among different studies. Intrinsic differences in the pediatric population like differences in dietary intake, malnutrition, vitamin deficiency etc. may favor the presence of different yeast species. Interactions among *Candida* species exists that favor coexistence of two or more species (synergistic) or render presence of particular species unlikely (antagonistic). The carriage of *C. tropicalis* and that of *C. glabrata* appears mutually exclusive, while carriage of *C. albicans* favors the presence of *C. glabrata* [37]. More studies are needed to explore this further.

Among the Candidal isolates, *C. albicans* has shown the highest prevalence. This may be attributed to its capacity to form germ tubes, facilitating adhesion [7]. Other factors such as molecular adhesion and invasion into host cells, the secretion of hydrolases, the yeast-to-hypha transition, contact sensing and thigmotropism, biofilm formation, and phenotypic switching contribute to its pathogenic potential [45]. The adhesion of *C. albicans* to intact and denatured type I collagen was found to be significantly greater than those of other species and suggested that *C. albicans* possessed the ability to adhere specifically to extracellular matrix as compared to other *Candida* species [46].

Virulence of *Candida* species is a significant factor that contributes to its colonization, pathogenicity, and infection of tissues [45]. In the present study, *Candida* expressed virulence factors such as formation of germ tubes, hyphae, hydrolytic enzymes such as phospholipases and hemolysin. Phospholipase acts by degrading the cell membrane of tissues and epithelial cells. *Candida* acquires iron from host tissue for its metabolism, growth, and invasion during host infection by the enzyme called hemolysin. There are reports of a higher production of virulence factors such as phospholipase among NAC than *C. albicans* [47]. Similar results are found in our study as all the isolates (100%) of *C. tropicalis*, C. *guilliermondii*, *C. glabrata*, and C. *kyfer* showed phospholipase production whereas only 96% of *C. albicans* were positive for phospholipase. However in the present study, the factors such as hemolysin production, germ tube, and hyphae were seen exclusively in *C. albicans.*

6. Virulence markers of candida species

C. albicans is an opportunistic pathogenic microorganism that has developed several virulence factors facilitating the invasion of host tissues [48]. It has the ability to persist on mucosal surfaces of healthy individuals [49]. In the oral cavity, it resists the mechanical washing action of a relatively constant flow of saliva towards the esophagus which contributes to its colonization and pathogenicity [50]. Its adhesion to host epithelial cells and biomaterials, formation of germ tubes and hyphae, the production of hydrolytic enzymes such as proteinases and phospholipases, and hemolytic capacity contribute to its colonization, pathogenicity, and infection of tissues [51].

The production of virulence factors is associated with the ability of *Candida* to cause infections [52]. Hemolytic capacity is an important virulence factor, which allows fungi of the genus *Candida* to acquire iron from host tissues, which then is used by the fungus for metabolism, growth, and invasion during host infection [53]. Phospholipase enzyme digests the host cell membrane phospholipid, causing cell lysis and changes in the surface features that enhance adherence and consequent infection. The ability to switch between the yeast form and the filamentous form is also an important virulence factor seen in *C. albicans*.

In the present study, germ tube and hyphal formation, an important virulence factor was seen among all the isolates of *C. albicans*. Phospholipase production was seen among 92.8% of the isolates which is higher than the values obtained from the previous studies by Deepa et al. [54] on Candidal isolates from Oral Candidiasis patients (52.6%) and Udaylaxmi et al. [16] on children on age 5–10 years with dental caries (47.6%). However, the results of the present study are lesser than that of Ali Zarei Mahmoudabadi et al. [55] on *C. albicans* isolated from vagina and urine samples, where phospholipase production was seen to be 100%. The phospholipase acts by degrading the cell membrane of tissues and epithelial cells, and it is an important virulence factor in progression of dental caries.

Hemolysis was shown by 2% among the Candidal isolates in the present study, which is lesser than the previous studies conducted by Rossinni et al. [56], Deepa et al. [54], and Udaylaxmi et al. [9], where the hemolysin activity was seen among 92, 63.1, and 100% of the isolates, respectively. There could be varied reasons for this variation. *Candida* strains in HIV-infected individuals have increased expression of virulence attributes as suggested by the strongly positive hemolytic activity among HIV individuals [56]. There are various factors that influence the morphology of yeast and its virulence, such as environmental changes like glucose starvation, growth temperature, carbohydrate rich diet, and the presence of streptococci [57].

Ketoconazole is an antifungal imidazole compound that exhibits a significant activity against a broad range of superficial and systemic infections caused by pathogenic yeasts, dermatophytes, and filamentous fungi, including *C. albicans*. It inhibits respiration by inhibiting the activity of NADH oxidase at the mitochondrial level which is its primary site of action. It is known to stimulate phagocytosis and inhibit ergosterol biosynthesis which is a characteristic constituent of yeast cell membranes thus inhibiting the filamentous growth of *C. albicans* [10]. Hence, ketoconazole is taken as the standard antifungal agent in the present study and other antimicrobial agents were compared with it.

0.2% Chlorhexidine digluconate is commonly used as an antiseptic mouth rinse because of its wide spectrum of antimicrobial activity. It is capable of inhibiting candidal adhesion to biological and inert surfaces resulting in biofilm [11]. It acts as a fungicide by coagulating the nucleoproteins of the cell walls causing the escape of cytoplasmic components through the plasmalemma [3]. A significant antimicrobial activity was shown by chlorhexidine, in the present study, with a mean zone of inhibition of 21.8 mm, and the difference with that of ketoconazole was not statistically significant (P value 0.54).

Coconut oil is known to exhibit antimicrobial activity against *S. mutans* and *C. albicans*. It has a unique role in the diet as an important physically functional food and is composed of medium chain fatty acids (MCFs) like lauric acid, caprylic acid, myristic acid, capric acid, linoleic acid, oleic acid, stearic acid, and palmitic acid. Lauric acid constitutes majority of MCFs in coconut oil and have similar beneficial effects as MCFs in mother's milk [58]. Monolaurin and other medium chain monoglycerides are shown to have the capacity to alter microbial cell walls, penetrate and disrupt cell membranes, and inhibit enzymes involved in energy production and nutrient transfer, leading to the death of the bacteria [59]. In the present study, coconut oil has shown antifungal activity that is comparable to that of ketoconazole. Previous studies have shown *C. albicans* to be highly susceptible to coconut oil [60], especially to the lauric acid of coconut oil [61].

Probiotics are live micro-organisms which, in adequate amounts, confer a health benefit to the host. Use of probiotics to replace cariogenic bacteria with noncariogenic beneficial microflora has shown promising results. Taking probiotics in cheese is found to reduce the prevalence of *C. albicans* [62]. In the present study, *C. albicans* was found to be susceptible to probiotics.

7. Conclusion

In the present study, the Candidal carriage among the children with dental caries was found to be 84%. In addition to *C. albicans*, non albicans *Candida* such as *C. tropicalis*, *C. guilliermondii*, *C. krusei*, *C. glabrata*, and *C. kyfer* were isolated from the teeth in children with dental caries which indicate its role in the production of dental caries. Various virulence factors such as phospholipase, hemolysin, and germ tube formation seem to affect its pathogenicity. This study scientifically proves the antifungal activity of chlorhexidine, coconut oil, and probiotics. The antifungal activity of coconut oil is found to be higher than that of probiotics against *C. albicans*.

However, further studies emphasizing the various other virulence factors such as proteinase production and phenotypic switching responsible for the virulence of the non albicans *Candida* need to be researched. Further studies must be carried out to determine the antimicrobial efficacy, the MIC, and MFC of these agents and more clinical studies have to be conducted to validate the same.

Acknowledgements

I acknowledge the support of Dr. Faial CP, Dr. Chandhru TP, Kannur Dental College and Dr. Shyamala R, Kannur Medical College, Anjarakandy towards this work.

Conflict of interest

I declare there is no conflict of Interest.

Author details

M.S. Beena
Master of Dental Surgery (MDS), Pediatric and Preventive Dentistry, Kerala University of Health Sciences, Kerala, India

*Address all correspondence to: beenamol40@yahoo.in

References

[1] Heymann HO, Swift EJ, Ritter AV, Sturdevant CM. Sturdevant's art and science of operative dentistry. In: Dental Caries: Etiology, Clinical Characteristics, Risk Assessment, and Management. 6th ed. St. Louis, Mo: Elsevier/Mosby; 2013. pp. 41-88

[2] Signoretto C, Burlacchini G, Faccioni F, Zanderigo M, Bozzola N, Canepari P. Support for the role of Candida spp. in extensive caries lesions of children. New Microbiologica. 2009;**32**:101-107

[3] Shino B, Peedikayil FC, Jaiprakash SR, Bijapur GA, Kottayi S, Jose D. Comparison of antimicrobial activity of Chlorhexidine, coconut oil, probiotics, and ketoconazole on *Candida albicans* isolated in children with early childhood caries: An in vitro study. Scientifica. 2016;**2016**:7061587. DOI: 10.1155/2016/7061587

[4] Klinke T, Kneist S, de Soet JJ, Kuhlisch E, Mauersberger S, Forster A, et al. Acid production by oral strains of Candida albicans and lactobacilli. Caries Research. 2009;**43**:83-91

[5] FragkouS,BalasouliC,TsuzukibashiO, ArgyropoulouA,MenexesG,KotsanosN, etal.Streptococcusmutans,Streptococcus sobrinus and Candida albicans in oral samples from caries-free and caries-active children. European Archives of Paediatric Dentistry. 2016;**17**:367-375

[6] Beena MS, Peedikayil FC, GufranAfmed MB, Chandru TP, Soni K, Dhanesh N. Comparison of Candida species isolated from children with and without early childhood caries: A descriptive cross-sectional study. Journal of the Indian Society of Pedodontics and Preventive Dentistry. 2017;**35**:296-300

[7] Nikawa H, Yamashiro H, Makihira S, Nishimura M, Egusa H, Furukawa M, et al. Invitro cariogenic potential of Candida albicans. Mycoses. 2003;**46**:471-478

[8] Barberi DDSAV, Vicente VA. Analysis of the in vitro adherence of Streptococcus mutans and Candida albicans. Brazilian Journal of Microbiology. 2007;**38**:624-631

[9] Udayalaxmi J, Shenoy N. Comparison between biofilm production, phospholipase and haemolytic activity of different species of Candida isolated from dental caries lesions in children. Journal of Clinical and Diagnostic Research: JCDR. 2016;**10**(4):DC21

[10] Uno J, Shigematsu ML, Arai T. Primary site of action of ketoconazole on Candida albicans. Antimicrobial Agents and Chemotherapy. 1982;**21**(6):912-918. DOI: 10.1128/aac.21.6.912

[11] Ellepola ANB, Samaranayake LP. Adjunctive use of chlorhexidine in oral candidosis: A review. Oral Diseases. 2001;7:11-17

[12] DebMandal M, Mandal S. Coconut (*Cocos nucifera L.: Arecaceae*): In health promotion and disease prevention. Asian Pacific Journal of Tropical Medicine. 2011;**4**(3):241-247

[13] Ashwell M. Concepts of functional foods Brussels: International Life Sciences Institute Europe. 2002

[14] Price MF, Wilkinson ID, Gentry LO. Plate method for detection of phospholipase activity in Candida albicans. Sabouraudia. 1982;**20**(1):7-14

[15] De Carvalho FG, Parisotto TM, Hebling J, Spolidorio LC, Spolidorio DM. Presence of Candida spp. in infants oral cavity and its association with early childhood caries.

Brazilian Journal of Oral Sciences. 2007;**1**:1249-1253

[16] Xiao J, Moon Y, Li L, Rustchenko E, Wakabayashi H, Zhao X, et al. Candida albicans carriage in children with severe early childhood caries (S-ECC) and maternal relatedness. PLoS One. 2016;**11**(10):e0164242

[17] Tinanoff N, O'sullivan DM. Early childhood caries: Overview and recent findings. Pediatric Dentistry. 1997;**19**:12-16

[18] Cannon RD, Chaffin WL. Oral colonization by Candida albicans. Critical Reviews in Oral Biology and Medicine. 1999;**10**(3):359-383

[19] Featherstone JD. The science and practice of caries prevention. Journal of the American Dental Association. 2000;**131**(7):887-899

[20] de Carvalho FG, Silva DS, Hebling J, Spolidorio LC, Spolidorio DM. Presence of mutans streptococci and Candida spp. in dental plaque/dentine of carious teeth and early childhood caries. Archives of Oral Biology. 2006;**51**(11):1024-1028

[21] Samaranayake LP, Hughes A, Weetman DA, MacFarlane TW. Growth and acid production of Candida species in human saliva supplemented with glucose. Journal of Oral Pathology & Medicine. 1986;**15**(5):251-254

[22] Manavathu EK, Dimmock JR, Vashishtha SC, Chandrasekar PH. Proton-pumping-ATPase-targeted antifungal activity of a novel conjugated styryl ketone. Antimicrobial Agents and Chemotherapy. 1999;**43**(12):2950-2959

[23] Allen CM, Saffer A, Meister RK, Beck FM, Bradway S. Comparison of a lesion inducing isolate and a non lesional isolate of Candida albicans in an immunosuppressed rat model of oral candidiasis. Journal of Oral Pathology & Medicine. 1994;**23**(3):133-139

[24] Hossain H, Ansari F, Schulz-Weidner N, Wetzel WE, Chakraborty T, Domann E. Clonal identity of Candida albicans in the oral cavity and the gastrointestinal tract of pre-school children. Oral Microbiology and Immunology. 2003;**18**(5):302-308

[25] Jose T, Thomas A, Pidamale R, Mhambrey S, Shetty SB. Research article. Correlation between C. albicans, S. mutans, S. sanguinis and lactobacillus in ECC, S-ECC and caries free children. International Journal of Recent Scientific Research. 2014;**5**(2):352-356

[26] Thomas A, Mhambrey S, Chokshi K, Chokshi A, Jana S, Thakur S, et al. Association of Oral Candida albicans with severe early childhood caries-a pilot study. Journal of Clinical and Diagnostic Research: JCDR. 2016;**10**(8):ZC109

[27] Maijala M, Rautemaa R, Järvensivu A, Richardson M, Salo T, Tjäderhane L. Candida albicans does not invade carious human dentine. Oral Diseases. 2007;**13**(3):279-284

[28] Peretz B, Mazor Y, Dagon N, Bar-Ness GR. Candida, mutans streptococci, oral hygiene and caries in children. The Journal of Clinical Pediatric Dentistry. 2011;**36**(2):185-188

[29] Ratson T, Greenstein RB, Mazor Y, Peretz B. Salivary Candida, caries and Candida in toothbrushes. The Journal of Clinical Pediatric Dentistry. 2012;**37**(2):167-170

[30] Şen BH, Safavi KE, Spångberg LS. Colonization of Candida albicans on cleaned human dental hard tissues. Archives of Oral Biology. 1997;**42**(7):513-520

[31] O'Donnell LE, Millhouse E, Sherry L, Kean R, Malcolm J, Nile CJ,

et al. Polymicrobial Candida biofilms: Friends and foe in the oral cavity. FEMS Yeast Research. 2015;**15**(7):fov077

[32] Hodson JJ, Craig GT. The incidence of Candida albicans in the plaques of teeth of children. Journal of Dentistry. 1972;**22**(8):296-301

[33] Rozkiewicz D, Daniluk T, Zaremba ML, Cylwik-Rokicka D, Stokowska W, Pawińska M, et al. Oral Candida albicans carriage in healthy preschool and school children. Advances in Medical Sciences. 2005;**51**:187-190

[34] Devi LS, Maheshwari M. Speciation of Candida species isolated from clinical specimens by using Chrom agar and conventional methods. International Journal of Scientific and Research Publications. 2014;**4**:1-5

[35] Moreira D, Spolidório DM, Rodrigues JA, Boriollo MF, Pereira CV, Rosa EA, et al. Candida spp. biotypes in the oral cavity of school children from different socioeconomic categories in Piracicaba-SP, Brazil. Pesquisa Odontológica Brasileira. 2001;**15**(3):187-195

[36] Martins AC, Maluf ML, Svidzinski TI. Prevalence of yeast species in the oral cavity and its relationship to dental caries. Acta Scientiarum: Health Sciences. 2011;**33**(1):107-112

[37] Al-hebshi NN, Abdulhaq A, Quadri MF, Tobaigy FM. Salivary carriage of Candida species in relation to dental caries in a population of Saudi Arabian primary school children. The Saudi Journal for Dental Research. 2015;**6**(1):54-59

[38] Al-Hebshi NN, Al-Maswary EA, Al-Hammadi ZO, Ghoname N. Salivary Candida species carriage patterns and their relation to caries experience among yemeni children. Oral Health & Preventive Dentistry. 2015;**13**:41-49

[39] Cortelli SC, Junqueira JC, da Silva FI, Ito CY, Cortelli JR. Correlation between Candida spp. and DMFT index in a rural population. Brazilian Journal of Oral Sciences. 2015;**5**(17):1007-1011

[40] Jabra-Rizk MA, Torres S, Rambob I, Meiller T, Grossman L, Minah G. Prevalence of oral Candida species in a North American pediatric population. The Journal of Clinical Pediatric Dentistry. 2007;**31**(4):260-263

[41] Al-Ahmad A, Auschill TM, Dakhel R, Wittmer A, Pelz K, Heumann C, et al. Prevalence of Candida albicans and Candida dubliniensis in caries-free and caries-active children in relation to the oral microbiota—A clinical study. Clinical Oral Investigations. 2015;**23**:1-9

[42] Lozano Moraga CP, Rodríguez Martínez GA, Lefimil Puente CA, Morales Bozo IC, Urzúa Orellana BR. Prevalence of Candida albicans and carriage of Candida non-albicans in the saliva of preschool children, according to their caries status. Acta Odontologica Scandinavica. 2016;**27**:1-6

[43] Erköse G, Erturan Z. Oral Candida colonization of human immunodeficiency virus infected subjects in Turkey and its relation with viral load and CD4+ T-lymphocyte count. Mycoses. 2007;**50**(6):485-490

[44] Samaranayake L. Commensal oral Candida in Asian cohorts. International Journal of Oral Science. 2009;**1**(1):2

[45] Mayer FL, Wilson D, Hube B. Candida albicans pathogenicity mechanisms. Virulence. 2013;**4**:119-128

[46] Makihira S, Nikawa H, Tamagami M, Hamada T, Nishimura H,

Ishida K, et al. Bacterial and Candida adhesion to intact and denatured collagen in vitro. Mycoses. 2002;**45**:389-392

[47] Butola R, Agwan V, Thakuria B, Madan M. A comparative study of virulence factors in clinical isolates of Candida species. International Journal of Current Microbiology and Applied Sciences. 2015;**4**:716-722

[48] Schaller M, Borelli C, Korting HC, Hube B. Hydrolytic enzymes as virulence factors of Candida albicans. Mycoses. 2005;**48**(6):365-377

[49] Bhat V. Prevalence of Candida associated denture stomatitis (CADS) and speciation of Candida among complete denture wearers of south west coastal region of Karnataka. Microbiology. 2013;**7**:8

[50] Noumi E, Snoussi M, Hentati H, Mahdouani K, Del Castillo L, Valentin E, et al. Adhesive properties and hydrolytic enzymes of oral Candida albicans strains. Mycopathologia. 2010;**169**(4):269-278

[51] Sitheeque MA, Samaranayake LP. Chronic hyperplastic candidosis/candidiasis (Candidal leukoplakia). Critical Reviews in Oral Biology and Medicine. 2003;**14**(4):253-267

[52] Aher CS. Species distribution, virulence factors and antifungal susceptibility profile of Candida isolated from Oropharyngeal lesions of HIV infected patients. International Journal of Current Microbiology and Applied Sciences. 2014;**3**(1):453-460

[53] Almeida RS, Wilson D, Hube B. Candida albicans iron acquisition within the host. FEMS Yeast Research. 2009;**9**(7):1000-1012

[54] Deepa K, Jeevitha T, Michael A. In vitro evaluation of virulence factors of Candida species isolated from oral cavity. Journal of Microbiology and Antimicrobials. 2015;**7**(3):28-32

[55] Mahmoudabadi AZ, Zarrin M, Miry S. Phospholipase activity of Candida albicans isolated from vagina and urine samples. Jundishapur Journal of Microbiology. 2010;**3**(4):169-173

[56] Rossoni RD, Barbosa JO, Vilela SF, Jorge AO, Junqueira JC. Comparison of the hemolytic activity between C. albicans and non-albicans Candida species. Brazilian Oral Research. 2013;**27**(6):484-489

[57] Holmes AR, Cannon RD, Jenkinson HF. Interactions of Candida albicans with bacteria and salivary molecules in oral biofilms. Journal of Industrial Microbiology. 1995;**15**(3):208-213

[58] Peedikayil FC. Is coconut oil good for oral health? A review. Journal of Health Research and Review. 2019;**6**:1-4

[59] Verallo-Rowell VM, Dillague KM, Syah, Tjundawan BS. Novel antibacterial and emollient effects of coconut and virgin olive oils in adult atopic dermatitis. Dermatitis. 2008;**19**(6):308-315

[60] Ogbolu DO, Oni AA, Daini OA, Oloko AP. In vitro antimicrobial properties of coconut oil on Candida species in Ibadan, Nigeria. Journal of Medicinal Food. 2007;**10**(2):384-387

[61] Devan K, Peedikayil FC, Kottayi S, Dhanesh N, Sursh KR. Antimicrobial efficacy of mdium chain fatty acids as root canal irrigants:An invitro study. Journal of the Indian Society of Pedodontics and Preventive Dentistry. 2019;**37**:258-264

[62] Hatakka K, Ahola AJ, Yli-Knuuttila H, et al. Probiotics reduce the prevalence of oral candida in the elderly—A randomized controlled trial. Journal of Dental Research. 2007;**86**(2):125-130

Chapter 4

Understanding Oral Diseases: Exploring Opportunities from Filipino Oral Microbiome Research

Marilen P. Balolong and Michael Antonio F. Mendoza

Abstract

The human mouth houses the second most diverse microbial community in the body, with almost 700 species of bacteria colonizing the hard surfaces of teeth and the soft tissues of the oral mucosa. To compete in the relatively exposed oral cavity, resident microbes must avoid being replaced by newcomers. This selective constraint, coupled with pressure on the host to cultivate a beneficial microbiome, has rendered a commensal oral microbiota that displays colonization resistance, protecting the human host from invasive species, including pathogens. Current control of dental plaque-related diseases is non-specific and is centered on the removal of plaque by mechanical means. Several new methods based on the modulation of the microbiome that aim at maintaining and re-establishing a healthy oral ecosystem have been developed and has greatly expanded our knowledge of the composition and function of the oral microbiome in health and disease. Promoting a balanced microbiome is therefore important to effectively maintain or restore oral health. This review provides an updated body of knowledge on oral microbiome in health and disease and discusses the implications for modern-day oral healthcare. Filipino Oral Microbiome Research to develop a policy framework for microbiome-based management of dental diseases and opportunities will be discussed.

Keywords: oral microbiome, dysbiosis, modulation, systemic diseases, oral health policy

1. Summary

Resident microorganisms have co-evolved and co-existed in our body in a mostly harmonious symbiotic relationship. The mouth, for instance, houses the second most diverse microbial community in the body, with almost 700 species of bacteria colonizing the hard surfaces of teeth and the soft tissues of the oral mucosa. Synergy and interaction of variable oral microorganisms help human body against invasion of undesirable stimulation outside. To compete in the relatively exposed oral cavity, resident microbes must avoid being replaced by newcomers. This selective constraint, coupled with pressure on the host to cultivate a beneficial microbiome, has rendered a commensal oral microbiota that displays colonization resistance, protecting the human host from invasive species, including pathogens. Perturbations of the oral microbiome through modern-day lifestyles can have detrimental consequences for our general and oral health. During dysbiosis, the equilibrium of the oral ecosystem is disrupted, allowing disease-promoting bacteria to manifest and cause conditions such as caries, gingivitis and periodontitis. In addition, rapid increases in carbohydrate consumption have disrupted the evolved homeostasis between the oral microbiota and dental health, as reflected by the high prevalence of dental caries. Development of novel modalities to prevent caries has been the subject of a breadth of research.

The current control of dental plaque-related diseases is nonspecific and is centered on the removal of plaque by mechanical means. The most prevalent oral diseases, dental caries and periodontal diseases, are microbiota-associated diseases. Due to this realization about the oral microbiome, several new methods based on the modulation of the microbiome that aim at maintaining and reestablishing a healthy oral ecosystem have been developed. Oral microbiomes play an important role in the human microbial community and human health. The use of recently developed molecular methods has greatly expanded our knowledge of the composition and function of the oral microbiome in health and disease. Studies in oral microbiomes and their interactions with microbiomes in variable body sites and variable health condition are critical in our cognition of our body and how to make effect on human health improvement. Through recent advances in technology, complexities of the oral microbiome have been slowly unraveled and new insights into its role during both health and disease are now made available. For practitioners and patients alike, promoting a balanced microbiome is therefore important to effectively maintain or restore oral health.

This chapter aims to give an update on our current knowledge of the oral microbiome in health and disease and to discuss implications for modern-day oral healthcare. More importantly, opportunities and future directions tapping Filipino Oral Microbiome Research will be explored toward developing a research-driven policy framework for microbiome-based management of dental diseases.

2. The oral microbiome: an overview

Humans have co-evolved with microorganisms [1], these commensals prevent colonization by exogenous microorganisms which translates their significant involvement in the normal development of the host defenses and gut mucosa, during the production of vitamin and energy as well as in the regulation of the cardiovascular system [2]. It was Antony van Leeuwenhoek who was first to identify oral microorganisms using his microscope, which is possibly the first account of oral microbiome [3], his "animalcules" [4].

The term "oral microbiome" has been coined to describe the microbial communities inhabiting the oral cavity behaving as a consortium involved in the modulation of various pathophysiological conditions of the host [5–7]. It is considered as the second most complex of the human body, after the gut-associated microbiome [8–10] with the average adult harboring about 50 to 100 billion bacteria represent about 200 predominant bacterial species [11]. Compared to other body sites, the oral microbiome is unique and readily accessible. However, there are only about 700 predominant taxa: 54% are cultivable and identified; 14% are cultivable but not yet identified, and the remaining 32% not even cultivated yet, the so-called "uncultivables" or phylotypes [5, 11–13]. These estimations are based on years of traditional identification of bacteria from cultural and phenotypic characterization studies, but mostly from identification of bacteria from culture-independent molecular studies using 16S rRNA gene comparative analyses [5, 14–17].

Figure 1 describes the transition and changes related microbiome profile in the mouth from sterility to oral disease state such as dental caries or systemic disease state. The fetus in the womb is usually sterile [18, 19]. The baby comes in contact with the microflora of the uterus and vagina of the mother during delivery, and later with the microorganisms of the atmosphere at birth [20]. The oral cavity of the newborn is considered sterile even though there is a high probability of contracting contaminants. Since the mouth is exposed to various microorganisms from the first feeding onward, this starts the process of acquiring the resident oral microflora [19]. Typically, the earliest colonizers of the tooth surface are commensal streptococci, such as *Streptococcus mitis, Streptococcus sanguinis, Streptococcus gordonii,* and other closely related taxa [21]. They antagonize transient microorganisms by producing by-products such as alkali, bacteriocins, and hydrogen peroxides. High abundances of these commensal streptococci are favored in dental plaque particularly in the absence of a carbohydrate-rich diet. This dominance is strongly associated with good dental health.

Historically, humans recorded two shifts in diet preference as influenced by the development of agriculture and by the industrial revolution [22] which favored the increase of carbohydrate consumption, particularly sucrose. With frequent consumption of carbohydrates such as sucrose coupled with poor oral hygiene, bacterial production of a certain glucan matrix is enhanced which can lead to the development of dental plaque, where other carbohydrate-related fermentation can continue. Due to the described changes that would result, perturbation of homeostasis of the oral microbiome can now lead to the development of dental caries, which is considered as the most common chronic disease worldwide, affecting 60–90% of children and adults even in industrialized countries [23].

It was previously mentioned that about 400 to 500 oral taxa have been detected in the subgingival crevice alone [14, 16] with the remaining taxa distributed to other oral habitats such as the tongue, tooth surface, buccal mucosa, tonsils, soft and hard palate, and lip vestibule [14, 24–26]. Although there is compositional variation between sample sites taken from the oral cavity, a 'core' microbiome in health has been identified [24, 25, 27]. Studies have also demonstrated that oral

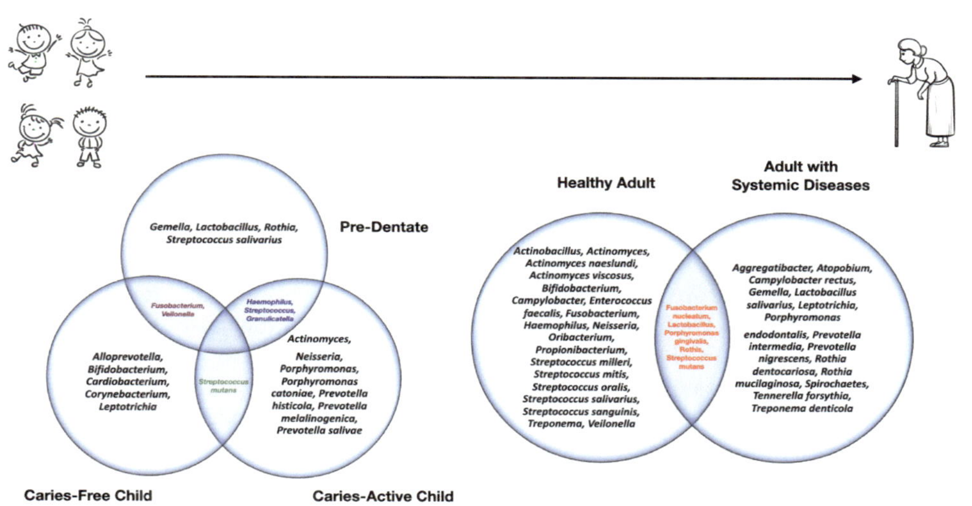

Figure 1.
Transition and changes related microbiome profile in the mouth from sterility to oral disease state such as dental caries or systemic disease state.

disease is not due to an isolated organism such as *Streptococcus mutans* causing caries, but is more polymicrobial in nature [5, 28, 29]. Studies have identified *Bifidobacterium, Veillonella, Granulicatetta, Scardovia, Fusobacterium, Prevotella* and *Actinomyces* as potential contributors to early childhood caries evidenced by their altered abundance in the caries microbiota [30].

Interestingly, there is a wide range of microorganisms that are said to inhabit the human oral cavity, including bacteria, fungi, viruses, archaea and protozoa which likewise contribute to influencing oral and systemic health [31]. Bacteria account for the main portion of oral microorganisms, and the major knowledge of the composition of oral bacteria comes from past culture-dependent methods, however, these data substantially underestimated the composition of the oral microbiome but development of culture-independent methods, particularly targeting 16S ribosomal RNA, offered expanded awareness of the great richness and diversity of the oral microbiome [31]. Fungi are present widely in the oral cavity not only as opportunistic pathogens of the elderly and immune-compromised but may also be present as members of the healthy oral microbiota [32]. Archaea constitutes only a minor part of the oral microbiome and is restricted to limited species [33, 34] observed in healthy subjects, but their prevalence and numbers are elevated in individuals with periodontitis [6]. Most viruses in the mouth are related to diseases including herpes simplex virus, human papilloma virus [35] and HIV infection indirectly related to observed oral manifestations, such as oral candidiasis, oral hairy leukoplakia, linear gingival erythema and necrotizing ulcerative periodontitis, and Kaposi's sarcoma [36].

The salivary or oral microbiome has been the target of interest for its diagnostic and prognostic value [37]. Since the commensal microbiome has an important role in the maintenance of oral and systemic health, altering its delicate balance may lead to the development of certain oral pathologies such as cavities endodontic disease, periodontal diseases, osteitis and tonsillitis [38–40] as well as various systemic diseases including cardiovascular disease [41], obesity [42–43], heart disease [44], diabetes [45], pediatric Crohn's Disease [46], pancreatic cancer [47], colon carcinoma [48], and even psychiatric disorders [49]. Studies during the last decade focused on the management and prevention of dental caries by modulating oral microbiome [37, 50]. However, it is yet to be established if there is a causal relationship between the oral microbiome and these systemic disorders. This battleground represents a significant opportunity for intervention and subsequent prevention of caries.

3. Methods employed in studying the oral microbiome: from "culturomics" to whole genome sequencing

Tables 1 and **2** show a comprehensive list of methods used in the study of oral microbiome from culture-dependent method to whole genome sequencing and OMICS. The relevant findings from the studies that utilized the various methods are also presented. Historically, as guided by Koch's postulates, cultivable bacterial taxa associated with various oral diseases were identified using culture-dependent methodologies such as microscopy, biochemical and other phenotypic tests, growth conditions, sugar utilization, and antibiotic sensitivity. However, this approach has presented various limitations when it comes to describing the actual diversity of the oral microbiome, or the so-called "great plate anomaly" [94, 95] and is unable to fully characterize complexity of bacterial communities such as those found in the oral cavity [60, 96].

Methods to study oral microbiome	Studies that have utilized the given methods	Important findings
Culture-Dependent Approach: "Culturomics"		
Heart Infusion Blood Agar (with menadione) Mitis Salivarius Medium (MS)	[51]	The cultivation on rich medium under anaerobic conditions, they investigated the overall composition of the microbiota of saliva, dental plaque, the gingival crevice, the cheeks, and the tongue dorsum They found organisms such as *Corynebacterium* spp., *Actinomyces* spp., and *Streptococcus sanguinis* colonizing teeth, treponemes in the gingival crevice, and *Streptococcus salivarius* on the tongue
MM10 Sucrose Medium MSB (MS + 20% sucrose, 0.2 U/ml bacitracin) Medium	[52]	Significant association between plaque levels of *S. mutans* and caries Saliva samples tended to have low levels of *S. mutans* and were equivocal in demonstrating a relationship between I and caries
MM10 Sucrose Medium MSB Medium LBS Medium	[53]	Clinical decay can occur in a few instances in the absence of detectable *S. mutans*, as was observed in the fissures high in lactobacilli
Trypticase Soy Broth (TSB) with 1% glucose	[54]	*Streptococcus mutans, Lactobacillus casei* and *Streprococcus faecalis* showed greater acid tolerance than strains of *Streptococcus sanguis, Streptococcus salivarius, Streptococcus mitis* and *Actinomyces viscosus* Species of plaque bacteria most closely associated with the initiation or progression of dental caries are more aciduric than non-cariogenic species
MSB medium GSTB medium (5% glucose, 5% sucrose, telurite, and bacitracin) TYCSB medium (tryptone, yeast extract, cysteine, sucrose, and bacitracin)	[55]	Early culture-based studies had shown that enamel caries was associated with increases in the numbers and proportions of mutans streptococci
Blood agar BM Medium	[56]	If such conditions of low pH are repeated on a regular basis, then the acidogenic/aciduric species are eventually able to increase their proportions and drive the plaque pH even lower, outcompeting the beneficial species
Tidd Hewitt Broth	[57]	There is heterogeneity in terms of expression of attributes among clinical strains belonging to a species, so that some strains of mutans streptocococci can be less acidogenic than isolates of other streptococcal species Emphasizes the need for detailed species and biovar identification of oral streptococci and for recognition of the significant physiological differences that occur within single species
BM Medium BMHGM Medium (BM supplemented with hog gastric mucin)	[58]	If such conditions of low pH are repeated on a regular basis, then the acidogenic/aciduric species are eventually able to increase their proportions and drive the plaque pH even lower, outcompeting the beneficial species

Methods to study oral microbiome	Studies that have utilized the given methods	Important findings
MTPY Medium TYCSB Medium	[59]	A total of 424 bifidobacteria were identified and these were *Bifidobacterium dentium*, *Parascardovia denticolens*, *Scardovia inopicata*, *Bifidobacterium longum*, *Scardovia* genomosp. C1 and *Bifidobacterium breve* Suggested that bifidobacteria may play a role in the progression of occlusal caries lesions in both children and adults Recent culture-based studies have correlated more diverse communities of bacteria with caries, including reporting on the association of *Actinomyces* and *Bifidobacterium* species with lesions, often with mutans streptococci comprising a relatively small percentage of the microbiota at diseased sites
BHI + HK Medium FAA Medium BUA medium	[5]	The human oral cavity contains a number of different habitats, including the teeth, gingival sulcus, tongue, cheeks, hard and soft palates, and tonsils, which are colonized by bacteria More than 700 prokaryotic taxa have been detected in the oral cavity, many of which cannot be isolated by common culture methods *Actinobacteria*, *Bacteroidetes*, *Chlamydiae*, *Chloroflexi*, *Euryarchaeota*, *Firmicutes*, *Fusobacteria*, *Proteobacteria*, *Spirochaetes*, SR1, *Synergistetes*, *Tenericutes*, and TM7
Cooked Meat Medium (CMM) CMM with mucin and serum Blood Agar	[60]	Cultivation of a *Synergistetes* strain representing a previously uncultivated strain from Subgingival plaque
Blood Agar MacConkey's Medium Chapman's Plate Growth Medium Chromagar-Candida	[61]	Samples deriving from oral cavity swabs, cultures, and *in vitro* tests showed the presence of various microorganisms belonging to different genera, species, and strains of bacteria, protozoans, and fungi in patient groups analyzed The pretreatment examination of oral cavity microbiota may be helpful in a preventive approach to the spread of infectious microorganisms, which may be etiological agents of human opportunistic infections and risk factors for treatment complications, particularly dangerous for older adults

Table 1.
Comprehensive list of methods used in the study of oral microbiome from culture-dependent methods to whole genome sequencing and OMICS. The relevant findings from the studies that utilized the methods are also presented.

Conventional cultivation of oral bacteria samples requires taking an appropriate sample, transferring the sample to an appropriate medium for transportation, and followed by correct storage following collection. Dispersion and plating the bacteria onto various culture media in the laboratory will then follow. The bacteria are then isolated and characterized by their colony morphologies (appearance) and biochemical testing. Species which do not grow are naturally "overlooked". One of the major challenges facing oral microbiology is the ability to culture the yet-to-be cultivated 32% of oral species. Furthermore, current knowledge existing about

Culture-Independent Approach: Pre-Next Generation Sequencing Era to Whole Genome Sequencing		
Studies that have utilized culture-independent methods	**Methods used**	**Important findings**
[14]	ABI Prism cycle sequencing kit	Highly common genera in various regions of cavity: *Gemella, Granulicatella, Streptococcus*, and *Veillonella*
[62]	16S ribosomal RNA genes polymerase chain reaction (PCR)	Tumor specimens: *Exiguobacterium oxido-tolerans, Prevotella melaninogenica, Staphylococcus aureus, Veillonella parvula* Non-tumor specimens: *Moraxella osloensis, Prevotella veroralis, Actinomyces* **Oral squamous cell carcinoma*
[63]	Comparative 16S rRNA gene sequencing and QPCR	Dental Plaque: Microbial community is dominated by *Streptococci* (66%) followed by *Actinomyces* (6%)
[64]	16S ribosomal RNA genes polymerase chain reaction (PCR) Restriction fragment length polymorphism 16S ribosomal RNA gene sequencing	*L. salivarius* was more prevalent in children with moderate to high caries prevalence compared with children with low caries prevalence, while *L. fermentum* was the most predominant species in all study groups. Genetic heterogeneity of *Lactobacillus* species was found among the children and those with high caries prevalence tended to be colonized with more than one clonal type *L. salivarius* may be a putative caries pathogen among preschool Thai children
[27]	454 Pyrosequencing FLX system	Dental surfaces, cheek hard palate, tongue and saliva: *Firmicutes*: *Streptococcus, Veillonellaceae, Granulicatella* *Proteobacteria*: *Neisseria, Haemophilus* *Actinobacteria*: *Corynebacterium, Rothia, Actinomyces* *Bacteroidetes*: *Prevotella, Capnocytophaga, Porphyromonas*
[65]	Sanger Sequencing	Gingiva: 247 species-level phylotypes and nine bacterial phyla
[5]	ABI Prism cycle sequencing kit	Various Regions of the Oral Cavity: A total of 619 taxa in 13 phyla *Actinobacteria, Bacteroidetes, Chlamydiae, Chloroflexi, Euryarchaeota, Firmicutes, Fusobacteria* *Proteobacteria, Spirochaetes*, SR1, *Synergistetes, Tenericutes*, and TM7
[60]	Fluorescent *in situ* Hybridization (FISH) Quantitative PCR (Q-PCR)	*Synergistetes* W090/OTU 6.2 to be prevalent and 'abundant' in both periodontally healthy subjects and those with chronic periodontitis, which would suggest that this bacterium is a commensal, endogenous to the oral cavity
[66]	454 Pyrosequencing FLX system	Supragingival and subgingival plaques: Five major phyla are *Bacteroidetes,*

Culture-Independent Approach: Pre-Next Generation Sequencing Era to Whole Genome Sequencing		
Studies that have utilized culture-independent methods	**Methods used**	**Important findings**
		Actinobacteria, Firmicutes, Proteobacteria and *Fusobacteria*
[67]	Arbitrarily primed PCR (AP-PCR) Chromosomal DNA fingerprinting DGGE	Ascertained the role of lactobacilli in the caries process Found seven LB species in the oral cavity of the subjects: *L. vaginalis, L. oris, L. gasseri, L. salivarius, L. fermentum, L. rhamnosus* and *L. casei*.
[68]	16S rRNA-based microarray and PCR	Several species, including *S. wiggsiae* and *S. exigua*, are associated with the ecology of advanced caries Successful treatment is accompanied by a change in the microbiota, and that severe early childhood caries is diverse, with influences from selected bacteria or from diet
[69]	454 GLX Titanium pyrosequencing	Results show a given bacterial consortium associated with cariogenic and non-cariogenic conditions, in agreement with the existence of a healthy oral microbiome and giving support to the idea of dental caries being a polymicrobial disease
[70]	454 Pyrosequencing using GS- FLX sequencer	Supragingival dental plaque: Healthy one: *Bacilli* and *GammaProteobacteria* dominated with specific association of *Rothia* and *Aggregatibacter* Diseased one: *Clostridiales* and *Bacteroidetes* dominated
[71]	Next generation sequencing of 16S rRNA gene DNA deduction	Data included 9 phyla, 16 classes, 26 orders, 55 families, and 111 genera (OUT was defined within 3% genetic difference) Detected approximately 29% more types of microbes than those detected from the same sample without using DNA deduction DNA deduction technique will lead to a better understanding of the diversity of the human oral microbiota
[72]	DGGE and Sanger sequencing	Oral Tissue: Six major phyla: *Firmicutes, Bacteroidetes Proteobacteria, Fusobacteria, Actinobacteria* and uncultivated TM7 with 80 bacterial species/phylotypes
[73]	PCR-DGGE	First study that provides a baseline profile of the oral microbial diversity in caries-free and caries-active Filipino adults using culture- independent techniques The caries-free group exhibited a more diverse microflora compared with its caries-active
[74]	Next generation sequencing 16S rRNA whole genome (454 FLX Titanium)	Saliva microbiomes in human population were featured by a vast phylogenetic diversity yet a minimal organismal core Caries microbiomes were significantly

Culture-Independent Approach: Pre-Next Generation Sequencing Era to Whole Genome Sequencing		
Studies that have utilized culture-independent methods	**Methods used**	**Important findings**
		more variable in community structure whereas the healthy ones were relatively conserved Abundance changes of certain taxa such as overabundance of *Prevotella* Genus distinguished caries microbiota from healthy ones Caries-active and normal individuals carried different arrays of *Prevotella* species No 'caries-specific' operational taxonomic units (OTUs) were detected, yet 147 OTUs were 'caries associated', that is, differentially distributed yet present in both healthy and caries-active populations
[75]	RNA-Seq Paired-end sequencing (Illumina HiSeq)	The bacteria changing activity during biofilm formation and after meal ingestion were person-specific Some individuals showed extreme homeostasis with virtually no changes in the active bacterial population after food ingestion, suggesting the presence of a microbial community which could be associated to dental health
[76]	16S pyrotag sequencing	Subgingival Plaque: Smokers: elevated number of *S. mutans, Lactobacillus sali varius* and commensal poor anaerobes
[77]	Roche 454 FLX sy	Swab: Significant reduction in *Firmicutes and Actinobacteria* while *Fusobacteria* count proportionally elevated in all oral cancer patients
[78]	Arbitrary-primed PCR (AP-PCR) Multi-locus Sequence Analysis (MLSA)	Develop a streamlined method for identifying strains of *S. oralis* and *S. mitis* from plaque samples so that they could be analyzed in a separate study devoted to low pH streptococci and caries Novel primer sets offer a convenient means of presumptive identification that will have utility in many studies where large scale, in-depth genomic analyses are not practical
[79]	RNA-Seq Paired-end sequencing (Illumina HiSeq)	There were similar levels of *Actinomyces* gene expression in both sound and carious root biofilms These bacteria can be commensal in root surface sites but may be cariogenic due to survival mechanisms that allow them to exist in acid environments and to metabolize sugars, saving energy
[80]	PhyloChip microarrays	Oral buccal mucosa: IBS-overweight participants showed decreased richness in the phylum *Bacteroidetes*

Culture-Independent Approach: Pre-Next Generation Sequencing Era to Whole Genome Sequencing		
Studies that have utilized culture-independent methods	**Methods used**	**Important findings**
[81]	454 Pyrosequencing FLX system	Oral rinse samples: 13 phyla having 122 genera Core microbiome constituted 7 phyla with 55 genera
[82]	454-pyrosequencing	Subgingival plaque: Diabetics: *Fusobacterium, Parvimonas, Peptostreptococcus* *Gemella, Streptococcus, Leptotrichia, Filifactor, Veillonella, TM7, Terrahemophilus and* elevated levels of *Capnocytophaga Pseudomonas, Bergeyella, Sphingomonas, Corynebacterium* *Propionibacterium*, and *Neisseria* in hyperglycemic individuals
[83]	Deep shotgun sequencing	Saliva from three pairs of populations of hunter-gatherers and traditional farmers living in close proximity in the Philippines Comparing these microbiomes with publicly available data from individuals living on a Western diet revealed that abundance ratios of core species were significantly correlated with subsistence strategy, with hunter-gatherers and Westerners occupying either end of a gradient of *Neisseria* against *Haemophilus*, and traditional farmers falling in between Species found preferentially in hunter-gatherers included microbes often considered as oral pathogens, despite their hosts' apparent good oral health
[84]	Next-generation sequencing of V3-V4 region of 16S rRNA gene (Illumina MiSeq)	Salivary microbiome was characterized in a group of children stratified by the Simplified Oral Hygiene Index (OHI-S) Twenty taxonomic groups (Seventeen genera, two families and one class; *Streptococcus*, *Veillonella*, *Gemellaceae*, *Prevotella*, *Rothia*, *Porphyromonas*, *Granulicatella*, *Actinomyces*, TM-7-3, *Leptotrichia*, *Haemophilus*, *Selenomonas*, *Neisseria*, *Megasphaera*, *Capnocytophaga*, *Oribacterium*, *Abiotrophia*, *Lachnospiraceae*, *Peptostreptococcus*, and *Atopobium*) were found in all subjects and constituted 94.5–96.5% of the microbiome Of these twenty genera, the proportion of *Streptococcus* decreased while *Veillonella* increased with poor oral hygiene status, *Veillonella dispar* and *Veillonella parvula* tended to be elevated in the Poor oral hygiene group
[85]	Next-generation sequencing of V4 region of 16S rRNA gene (Illumina MiSeq)	A comprehensive analysis of the oral microbiome identified *Granulicatella* and *Neisseria* as bacteria enriched in subjects with MetS and *Peptococcus* as bacteria abundant in healthy controls

Culture-Independent Approach: Pre-Next Generation Sequencing Era to Whole Genome Sequencing		
Studies that have utilized culture-independent methods	**Methods used**	**Important findings**
		Results support that local oral microbiota can be associated with systemic disorders The microbial biomarkers identified would aid in determination of which individuals develop chronic diseases from their MetS and contribute to strategic disease management
[86]	Next-generation sequencing of V1-V2 region of 16S rRNA gene (Illumina MiSeq)	*Porphyromonas*, *Treponema*, *Tannerella*, *Filifactor*, and *Aggregatibacter* were more abundant in patients with periodontal disease, whereas *Streptococcus*, *Haemophilus*, *Capnocytophaga*, *Gemella*, *Campylobacter*, and *Granulicatella* were found at higher levels in healthy controls
[87]	Fluorescence in situ hybridization and Confocal Laser Scanning Microscopy	Establishes *S. oralis* as commensal keeper of homeostasis in the biofilm by antagonizing *S. mutans*, thus preventing a caries-favoring dysbiotic state
[88]	Next-generation sequencing of V3-V4 region of 16S rRNA gene (Illumina MiSeq)	Interproximal-associated microbiota was found to be similar to already described bacterial communities in other mouth niches. *Streptoccocus, Veillonella, Rothia, Actinomyces, Neisseria, Haemophilus* and *Fusobacterium* were the most abundant genera in this oral region
[30]	Next-generation sequencing of V4-V5 region of 16S rRNA gene (Illumina MiSeq)	Distinct differences between the caries microbiota and saliva microbiota were identified, with separation of both salivary groups (caries-active and caries-free) The major phyla of the caries active dentinal microbiota were Firmicutes (median abundance value 33.5%) and Bacteroidetes (23.2%), with *Neisseria* (10.3%) being the most abundant genus, followed by *Prevotella* (10%). The caries-active salivary microbiota was dominated by Proteobacteria (median abundance value 38.2%) and Bacteroidetes (27.8%) with the most abundant genus being *Neisseria* (16.3%), followed by *Porphyromonas* (9.5%). Caries microbiota samples were characterized by high relative abundance of *Streptococcus mutans*, *Prevotella* spp., *Bifidobacterium* and *Scardovia* spp.
[89]	Next-generation sequencing of V3-V4 region of 16S rRNA gene (Illumina MiSeq)	Provides thorough knowledge of the microbiological etiology of elderly individuals with caries and is expected to provide novel methods for its prevention and treatment
[90]	Next-generation sequencing of V3-V4 region of 16S rRNA gene (Illumina MiSeq)	Decrease in commensal saliva bacteria were observed in all the body sizes when compared to normal weight children. Notably, the relative abundance of bacteria

Culture-Independent Approach: Pre-Next Generation Sequencing Era to Whole Genome Sequencing		
Studies that have utilized culture-independent methods	**Methods used**	**Important findings**
		related to, *Veillonella*, *Prevotella*, *Selenomonas,* and *Streptococcus* was reduced in obese children Body size–specific saliva microbiota profiles open new avenues for studying the potential roles of microbiota in weight development and management
[91]	Fluorescence in situ hybridization and Confocal Laser Scanning Microscopy	Investigated the impact of various *Fusobacterium* species on *in vitro* biofilm formation and structure in three different oral biofilm models namely a supragingival, a supragingival "feeding", and a subgingival biofilm model Study showed variations in the growing capacities of different fusobacteria within biofilms, affecting the growth of surrounding species and potentially the biofilm architecture
[92]	Next-generation sequencing of V4 region of 16S rRNA gene (Illumina MiSeq)	Adult oral microbiomes were predominantly impacted by oral health habits, while youth microbiomes were impacted by biological sex and weight status The oral pathogen *Treponema* was detected more commonly in adults without recent dentist visits and in obese youth Oral microbiomes from participants of the same family were more similar to each other than to oral microbiomes from non-related individuals
[8]	Whole Genome Sequencing Real-time quantitative PCR microarray	Sampled oral micro-habitat included tongue dorsum, hard palate, buccal mucosa, keratinized gingiva, supragingival and subgingival plaque, and saliva with or without rinsing. Each sampled oral niche evidenced a different microbial community, including bacteria, fungi, and viruses Oral rinse microbiome was more representative of the whole site-specific microbiomes, compared with that of saliva Healthy oral microbiome resistome included highly prevalent genes conferring resistance to macrolide, lincosamides, streptogramin, and tetracycline.
[93]	Next-generation sequencing of V3-V4 region of 16S rRNA gene (Illumina MiSeq)	A comparison of oral bacteriome between two groups revealed the dominance of acidogenic and aciduric bacteria in diabetics which suggested the involvement of these eubacteria in oral dysbacteriosis in diabetes mellitus Phylum Firmicutes (p-value = 0.024 at 95% confidence interval) was significantly more abundant among diabetic patients than among the controls

Culture-Independent Approach: Pre-Next Generation Sequencing Era to Whole Genome Sequencing		
Studies that have utilized culture-independent methods	**Methods used**	**Important findings**
		Acidogenic bacteria *Prevotella* (p-value = 0.024) and *Leptotrichia* (p-value = 1.5×10^{-3}); and aciduric bacteria *Veillonella* (p-value = 0.013) were found to be in higher abundance in diabetic patients

Table 2.
Comprehensive list to describe methods in the study of oral microbiome from culture-dependent methods to whole genome sequencing and OMICS + studies that have utilized hem through the years).

pathogens linked to oral diseases are based on bacterial communities that have somehow survived transportation in a sample, grew easily or rapidly in the laboratory, based on a culture method employed in the laboratory [96, 97] which seems to limited and fundamentally incomplete.

Resultant knowledge of oral microbial ecology and dynamics have enabled development of novel culture techniques that have somehow helped the cultivation of some strains including the provision of distinct conditions such as an anaerobic (oxygen-free) environment, incubation in a variety of temperatures, use of chemically-defined media containing specific amounts of nutrients, and even the use of cytokine networks and microbial co-colonizers [98, 99]. But despite these advances, still many organisms remained uncultivable due to several assumptions [98, 100] such as (1) they exist in obligate metabolic associations with other organisms; (2) since oral bacteria do not live in isolation but in complex communities called biofilms, they depend on synergies and antagonisms for growth, along with mutual reliance for growth and survival; and (3) the lack of essential nutrients, growth factors and/or signaling molecules, overfeeding conditions, lack of cross-feeding partners, culture media toxicity and disruption of bacterial quorum-sensing and other signaling systems or other reasons that remained to be undiscovered until now.

Cultivation remains the foundation of oral microbiology in characterizing phenotypically, identification, including physiology and pathogenicity of particular species. The proportion therefore of the so-called 'overlooked' bacteria that are responsible for a number of oral diseases [99] must be studied using molecular signatures in order to include a huge number of uncultivable species found in healthy and diseased sites in the human mouth and to better understand the many aspects of microbial dynamics in the oral cavity [95, 98, 101]. The development and advances in molecular techniques, therefore, can help enhance and enable the study of complex host-associated bacterial communities such as those in the oral cavity.

Watson and Crick's discovery of the DNA structure helped clarify the mechanism of base pairing and explained how genetic information is stored and copied in living organisms. This knowledge then led to the power to investigate microbial communities or individual cells from detection to identification to diversity profiling using molecular-based technologies. Molecular techniques have enabled a more in-depth investigation and have resulted in different and more focused approaches compared to cultivation [102].

Early high-throughput analytical approaches in studying microbial communities utilized the fragment size separation differences of the DNA such as the denaturing gradient gel electrophoresis (DGGE) and the restriction fragment length polymorphism (RFLP) methods which based findings on [103, 104] following amplification of target regions of interest through the polymerase chain reaction or PCR. These types of approach enabled analysis at the macro-level for microbial communities characterized by large shifts or variations in the population. DNA–DNA hybridization and DNA microarrays followed providing rapid assessment of specific bacterial associations in oral health and disease [105] with the use of hybridized DNA fragments and complementary probes arrayed on a glass slide for expression profiling [106].

The modern era of microbial genome analysis began in the early 2000s, with metagenomics and gene sequencing techniques [107]. The 16S rRNA gene is usually selected as the target gene because it comprises both variable and conserved regions, permitting the use of primers to conserved regions and more specific primers to amplify 16S rRNA genes from any source to discriminate between taxa [108, 109]. Bacterial taxa can be phylogenetically identified, whether they are cultivable or not-yet-cultivated, in a mixed population, e.g., plaque, by isolating DNA, amplification of universally conserved primers for 16S rRNA gene, a conserved gene of approximately 1500 bp, followed by cloning into *Escherichia coli*, and lastly Sanger sequencing [16] or the more modern next generation sequencing [110]. Among nine distinct hypervariable regions, V_1, V_2, V_3 and V_4 stretches are highly exploited sequences for studying microbial diversity due to their extreme variability; V_5 exhibits least variability [111] while V_{4-6} region is considered as the most reliable stretch that represents the entire length of 16S rDNA for studying the majority of bacterial phyla [110]. Currently, oral microbiome-based next generation sequencing analysis chiefly relies on primers of either V_{1-2} or V_{3-4} regions. These bits and pieces of 16S rDNA regions are capable enough of providing the entire picture of bacterial phyla present in a niche; however, ambiguous data obtained from various targeted variable regions cannot be ignored, and it demands a massive full- length sequencing of 16S rDNA region for its validation. Interestingly, the use of V_1 region has been linked to differentiating *Streptococci*, a pioneer of the oral cavity, while region V_2 is associated to accurately identify various phylotypes of Gram-negative *Porphyromonas* and *Fusobacterium* [111]. Furthermore, amplifying $V_{1-3 \text{ works best for}}$ *Streptococcus, Fusobacterium, Prevotella, Porphyromonas*, and *Bacteroides*, but the use of V_{4-6} region showed observed dominance of *Prevotella, Porphyromonas, Treponema, Enterococci* and *Campylobacter*-like oral inhabitants [112]. In the last decade, next generation sequencing methods have revolutionized the study of microbial diversity, and enabled large-scale sequencing projects to be completed in a few days or sometimes hours.

The use of universal bacterial primers for simultaneous analysis of a wide variety of bacteria in the oral microbiota is undeniably extensive. Some limitations related to its possible binding to the same conserved area of the 16S rRNA target population have been reported and cannot be ignored such as those linked to probable PCR competitive inhibition. In this scenario, the DNA of the predominant (major) bacterial species is much more likely to be amplified than DNA from bacteria that form a minority or small proportion of the overall mixed population which could lead (in theory) to the complete omission of the DNA of minority bacterial species from the analysis [113]. Amplification of the DNA species present in excess (competitor DNA) may result at the expense of the DNA species present in smaller amounts limiting the analysis to only the majority species present. To address this, Kuwamura and Kamiya [114] developed the "DNA deduction" approach where excess DNA of the majority bacterial species present in the target population is removed and the detection of minority bacterial members of the community is facilitated. This method was proved to be a useful technique to better understand the diversity and composition of the human oral microbiota since many researchers identify species based on 16S rRNA sequence information in studying the oral microbiota [115, 116]. Since a large number of good-quality sequences is required in order to construct a precise DNA database for use in human microbiota analyses for next generation sequencing, DNA deduction technique may offer improvement of the human microbiota database.

Molecular techniques based on next-generation sequencing (NGS) of the 16 rRNA gene of the bacterial genome, allowed analysis of the complexity of the bacterial component of the oral microbiome and has represented the standard for studying the composition of microbial communities by allowing differentiation of bacteria by sequencing the variable regions of the gene coding for the 16S ribosomal RNA (rRNA) which greatly improved our knowledge of the bacterial component of the oral microbiome [13, 117]. However, it does not usually provide sufficient information to resolve communities at the sub-species level, nor it can detect eukaryotic microorganisms and/or viruses. Instead, the species-level resolution obtained by NGS is not adequate for transmission studies or for exploring subspecies variation in disease association, and the oral microbiome includes also important non-bacterial components, including eukaryotic microbes (fungi, protozoa) and viruses [8]. For instance, reports on normal microbiome have been almost exclusively restricted to the bacteriome, and there are limited published findings on the mycobiome–fungal microbiome and on other microorganisms. To simultaneously characterize the presence and amount of all the microbial components potentially present in the oral cavity, the Whole Genome Sequencing (WGS) was introduced very recently [118, 119]. In whole genome sequencing, the entire DNA (genome) of a single microbial culture or a complex microbial population can now be sequenced to great depth allowing us to generate reference genomes (de novo assembly) as a resource for future studies or identify the composition of microbial community respectively (mapping back to a reference genome).

Another important aspect that may not also be addressed in depth is the issue related to antimicrobial resistance or AMR, very limited reports are available on resistome of the healthy oral microbiome [120, 121]. Since AMR is a growing concern, it would be useful to have data on the prevalence and type of drug resistance of the microbes composing the healthy oral microbiome, which might be very easily acquired and transmitted through aerosol and contact. Recently, Caselli et al. [8] provided comprehensive and detailed picture of the healthy oral microbiome as determined by WGS analysis, including also the drug-resistance features of the bacterial component. These findings further strengthened laboratory capabilities and added more areas for oral microbiome research to enable evidence-based oral diseases management in practice.

4. Impacts of oral microbiome to oral health (dental caries) and non-oral health (systemic diseases)

Oral microbiome data have accumulated in recent years and somehow slowly influences how we see management of oral diseases. During the last decade, studies have focused on the management and prevention of certain and disorders such as dental caries by modulating oral microbiome [37, 50]. Interestingly, some member of the oral microbiota has also been tagged as possible effective biosensors or biomarkers of oral or systemic diseases [84, 122]. In addition, the salivary or oral microbiome has been the target of interest for its diagnostic and prognostic value [37]. **Table 3** comprehensively lists the studies that supported the impacts of oral microbiome studies to both Oral and Non-Oral or Systemic Health.

Dental diseases are now viewed as a consequence of a deleterious shift in the balance of the normally stable resident oral microbiome. It is known that frequent

Oral microbiota derived from microbiome data	Associated disease status	References
Fusobacterium nucleatum	Periodontal disease	[123]
Eubacterium minutum *Prevotella intermedia*	Peri-implantitis	[124]
Haemophilus	Oral leukoplakia (mucosal disease)	[125]
Fusobacteria *Leptotrichia spp* *Campylobacter concisus*		[126]
Prevotella spp. *Lactobacillus* spp. *Dialister* spp. *Filifactor* spp.	Pathogenesis and progression of dental caries	[127]
Veillonella *Porphyromonas* *Streptococcus mutans*	Severe early childhood caries	[128]
Streptococcus *Porphyromonas* *Actinomyces*		Ma et al., 2015
Streptococcus *Prevotella* *Neisseria* *Haemophilus* *Veillonella* *Gemella*	Inflammatory Bowel Disease	[129]
Klebsiella spp.		Atarashi et al., 2017
Acinetobacter calcoaceticus *Atopobium rimae* *Clavibacter michiganensis subsp. tessellarius* *Bacillus mycoides* *Capnocytophaga gingivalis* *Citrobacter koseri* *Curtobacterium flaccumfaciens* *Delftia acidovorans* *Eikenella corrodens isolate* *Escherichia coli* *Enterococcus faecalis* *Lactobacillus gasseri* *Fusobacterium canifelinum, Fusobacterium naviforme, Fusobacterium nucleatum* ssp. 1 *nucleatum* *Gemella haemolysans, Gemella morbillorum* *Leptotrichia shahii* *Megasphaera micronuciformis* *Moraxella osloensis* *Ralstonia insidiosa, Ralstonia pickettii, Ralstonia solanacearum* *Rothia* *Novel Atopobium* *Olsenella uli* *Plantibacter flavus* *Propionibacterium acnes* *Parvimonas* *Peptostreptococcus micros, Peptostreptococcus stomatis* *Porphyromonas* *Prevotella melaninogenica* *Rhodococcus erythropolis* *Rothia mucilaginosa*	Oral Squamous Cell Carcinoma	[130] [131] [132] [72] [133] [134] [7]

Oral microbiota derived from microbiome data	Associated disease status	References
Slackia *Streptococcus gordoniii, Streptococcus salivarius, Streptococcus sanguinis* *Tepidimonas aquatica* *Thermus scotoductus*		
Porphyromonas gingivalis *Aggregatibacter actinomycetemcomitans* *Leptotrichia*	Pancreatic Cancer	[135] [136] [39]
Streptococcus	Pancreatic Ductal Adenocarcinoma	[137]
Rothia *Peptostreptococcus* *Fusobacterium* *Leptotrichia*	Pancreatic Head Cancer	[138]
Porphyromonas gingivalis	Gingival Squamous Cell Carcinoma	[139]
Rothia mucilaginosa *Lactobacillus gasseri* *Lactobacillus johnsonii* *Lactobacillus gavinalis* *Streptococcus salivarius* *Streptococcus vestibularis* *Fusobacterium nucleatum*	Head and Neck Squamous Cell Carcinoma	[140]
Rothia mucilaginosa *Capnocytophaga gingivalis* *Prevotella melininogenica* *Gemella morbillorum* *Granulicatella adiacens* *Streptococcus gordonii* *Streptoccus parasanguinis* *Stretococcus salivarius* *Fusobacterium nucleatum*	Oral Potentially Malignant Disorder	[141]
Gemella morbillorum	Keratocytic Odontogenic Tumor	[142]
Streptococcus *Fusobacterium*	Colorectal Carcinoma	[143]
Porphyromonas gingivalis *Prevotella* *Streptococcus*	Esophageal Squamous Cell Carcinoma	[144, 145]
Streptococcus	Gastric Adenocarcinoma	[146]
Prevotella melaninogenica *Fusobacterium*	Oral Cancer	[77]
Rothia mucilaginosa *Streptococus*	Oral Mobile Tongue Carcinoma	[147]
Actinobacillus actinomycetemcomitans *Tannerella forsythia* *Porphyromonas gingivalis* *Fusobacterium nucleatum* *Prevotella intermedia*	Alzheimer's disease	[148, 149]
Aggregatibacter *Neisseria* *Gemella* *Eikenella*	Diabetes	[150]

Oral microbiota derived from microbiome data	Associated disease status	References
Selenomonas *Actinomyces* *Capnocytophaga* *Fusobacterium* *Veillonella* *Streptococcus*		
Bacteroides forsythus *Campylobacter rectus*	Adverse pregnancy outcomes	[151]
Fusobacterium nucleatum		[152]
Lactobacillus salivarius	Rheumatoid arthritis	[153]
Veillonella *Prevotella* *Megasphaera* *Campylobacter*	Human Immunodeficiency Virus infection	[154]
Chryseomonas *Veillonella* *Streptococcus*	Atherosclerosis	[155]

Table 3.
Comprehensive list of studies supporting the impacts of Oral microbiome data (healthy or dysbiosis) to Oral and non-Oral health.

carbohydrate consumption or reduced saliva flow can lead to caries, and excessive plaque accumulation increases the risk of periodontal diseases. In general, increase in fermentable carbohydrates in the oral cavity or saliva, which is usually the case in diabetes, establishes a favorable environment for the microbes involved in dental caries [13]. However, reports have also described that shifts in the proportion of plaque microflora may not be directly caused by the mere availability of certain fermentable carbohydrates but rather, brought about by pH-mediated mediated reactions generated from carbohydrate metabolism [56]. Hence, it can be suggested that modifying metabolism of certain carbohydrates may result in slowing down the enrichment of cariogenic species, preventing development of caries. The excess uptake of carbohydrates leads to acid production due to fermentation of carbohydrates by many oral cavity inhabitants which disturbs the buffering capacity of saliva and hence results in tooth decay or dental caries.

Changes in environmental conditions brought about by poor oral hygiene may favor certain members of the oral microbiota and consequently serve as biomarkers for certain oral disease condition. Saliva and diet were observed to alter *Lactobacillus* abundance in the pulpal layer [156], and that low levels of *Lactobacillus* were linked to the degree and duration of pain and length of caries destruction. Moreover, poor oral hygiene status seems to be linked to anaerobic conditions in the salivary milieu, this condition inhibits growth of *Streptococcus* and favors the growth of *Veillonella* [153, 157, 158]. Salivary and plaque microbiome data also revealed that *Veillonella* was frequently found in subjects with caries or periodontal subjects, whether children or adults, with poor oral health and having caries or periodontitis [84]. Based on these findings, the proportion of *Veillonella* in salivary microbiome, therefore, can serve as a biological indicator for poor oral hygiene and caries in children and adults.

Oral microbial dysbiosis is also linked to oral inflammation and may contribute to systemic conditions through bacteremia [159]. It contributes to variable systemic diseases processing including gastrointestinal system diseases like inflammatory bowel disease, liver cirrhosis, pancreatic cancer, nervous system diseases like Alzheimer's disease, endocrine system diseases like diabetes, adverse pregnancy outcomes, obesity and polycystic ovary syndrome, immune system diseases like rheumatoid arthritis and HIV infection, and cardiovascular system diseases like atherosclerosis [160].

The dominant genera, *Streptococcus, Prevotella, Neisseria, Haemophilus, Veillonella* and *Gemella*, were found to largely contribute to dysbiosis observed in the salivary microbiota of IBD patients [129]. A growing interest regarding the variation of salivary microbiota between dental caries patients with comorbidities such as rheumatoid arthritis (RA) and atherosclerosis compared to healthy subjects. Alterations in the gut, dental or saliva microbiome distinguished individuals with RA from healthy controls, were correlated with clinical measures and could be used to stratify individuals on the basis of their response to therapy. It was observed that *Haemophilus* species seems to be depleted from saliva, dental plaque and fecal samples of RA patients but their numbers become normal upon standard RA treatment [153]. Interestingly, the levels of *Porphyromonas gingivalis*, *Treponema denticola*, *Tannerella forsythia* and *Prevotella intermedia* in the saliva, have been linked in lowering serum levels of high-density lipoproteins, which may be associated with an increased risk of atherosclerosis [122]. These findings also highlight the possibility of saliva-based screening as alternative to fecal samples in microbiologic studies of systemic diseases.

Microbes are believed to be released from the biofilm through the epithelium and spread systemically via the blood circulation, this is probably the reason why bacteria isolated from pancreatic tissues are believed to be possible members of the oral microbiome [161]. *Porphyromonas gingivalis* is an important bacterium that can be transferred from the mouth to gut in many diseases, including colon cancer, IBD, and diabetes [138]. This microorganism induces dysbiosis by impairing innate host defenses while promoting inflammatory responses in phagocytic cells. Since this microbe can disrupt the interaction between host microbiota and mucosa by modulating the innate immune system and signaling pathway enhancing high levels of inflammation in pancreatic cancer [162], it is believed to be a good candidate biosensor for early diagnosis of pancreatic cancer. Likewise, oral metabolome finds its application in determination of biomarkers in oral cancers [163]. An elevated rate of degradation of macromolecules was shown in metabolome profiling in periodontal disease. Shifts in metabolic profiles indicate survival of pathogens in given conditions.

Disruption of the oral microbiome leads to dysbiosis. Identifying the microbiome in health is the first step of human microbiome research, after which it is necessary to understand the role of the microbiome in the alteration of functional and metabolic pathways associated with diseased states [9]. Salivary microbiota composition and abundance were significantly associated with body size and dependent on gender; particularly notable was the decrease in the core bacteria in overweight and obese children [90]. Overweight and obese children are likely to stay obese into adulthood and develop diseases more frequently than normal weight children. Thus, the early identification of subjects at risk of developing obesity and the prevention of overweight and obesity is of great importance. As we increase our understanding of the interplay between the environment and the oral microbiome, it will become possible to identify new strategies to combat disease by actively promoting our natural microbiota and reducing the impact of the drivers of dysbiosis [164].

Future studies focusing on precision medicine and risk prediction for dental caries and even periodontitis may also be possible when changes in oral microbiota profiles in the salivary milieu may be made available. Previous studies have supported this which targeted subtypes or strains of specific bacterial species such as *Porphyromonas gingivalis* or *Aggregatibacter actinomycemcomitans* [165] in periodontits or *Streptococcus mutans* in caries [166] in predicting common oral health risks. Characterizing oral biofilms by metabolic activity rather than by listing the predominant species may also be considered as a logical approach when defining plaque biofilms in health and disease.

5. Novel microbiome-based approaches to prevention and treatment of dental caries

Traditional intervention methods to addressing dental diseases include mechanical debridement and antibiotic use. Mechanical means are non-specific and may remove beneficial bacteria in the process, more importantly, the microbial richness and biodiversity are also significantly decreased after mechanical debridement [167] which is not beneficial to overall oral health. Antibiotics on the other hand are designed to target specific pathogenic bacteria in animals and humans [168]. It was reported that the number of amoxicillin-resistant oral bacteria was significantly higher in young children with amoxicillin use than that of children without [169]. In view of the role of oral microorganisms in the causation and pathogenesis of oral and systemic diseases, it is crucial to improve oral protection against pathogens and maintain the dynamic equilibrium of the oral microecology. Understanding the interactions between the microbial communities is a key to combating oral pathogens. Novel strategies have been developed, such as the use of probiotics and prebiotics to address limitations of traditional intervention methods.

Probiotics are well-known in health promotion, they are "live microorganisms when administered in adequate amounts, confer a health benefit on the host" [170]. The mechanism of action of probiotics in the mouth is presumed to be similar to those observed in other parts of the body [171] which is to act mainly through these paths: competition with potential pathogens for nutrients or adhesion sites, killing or inhibition of growth of pathogens through production of bacteriocins or other products, improvement of intestinal barrier integrity and upregulation of mucin production, modulation of cell proliferation and apoptosis, and stimulation and modulation of the mucosal immune system [171, 172]. Oral probiotics should have specific characteristics to perform effectively including the ability to stick to and colonize oral tissue including hard, non-shedding surfaces and become a part of the biofilm [171, 173]. Additionally, they should not ferment sugars; otherwise, they will decrease pH and develop caries [171]. Probiotic methods have been studied to treat caries mainly by interfering with the oral colonization of cariogenic pathogens. Some strains that were used include *Lactobacillus casei* [174], *L. rhamnosus* GG [175], *L. rhamnosus, Bifidobacterium* [176], *Lactobacillus reuteri* [177], *B. animalis* [178], and *L. paracasei* [179], all of which have been verified to be able to decrease the number of cariogenic bacteria and thus, prevent dental caries.

Prebiotics, on the otherhand are poorly digested oligosaccharides and have been demonstrated to be an aid to complement probiotics in the treatment of oral diseases [172] by stimulating the growth and activity of beneficial bacteria and simultaneously inhibiting the growth and activity of potentially detrimental bacteria [172]. Some examples are Lactose, Inulin, Fructo oligosacccharides, Galactooligosaccharides and Xylooligosaccharides [180]. However, studies on prebiotic utilization seems limited and should be further investigated. Based on these findings, probiotics and prebiotics could be alternatives to prevent and cure bacterial diseases because they can reestablish an ecological balance or regain the biodiversity of oral microbiota in its early stages [181]. Prebiotics can drive beneficial changes in the oral microbiota and could increase resistance to dysbiosis and recovery of health. However, interaction between the oral microbiome and probiotics, as well as the exact mode of action of oral probiotics should be taken into serious consideration.

Other promising alternatives to control dental caries are the use of avirulent *S. mutans* produced by genetic engineering [182], which was designed to target glucosyltransferases and consequently inhibit biofilm formation [183].

The use of bacteriophage or phage is a virus that specifically targets and destroys disease-causing bacteria by invading bacterial cells [182], disrupting their metabolism and causing lysis such as phages against *Enterococcus faecalis* that showed reduction in bacterial viability in infected root canals [184]. Several targeted delivery systems have been designed and developed to treat oral diseases including nanoparticles [185–187].

Modulation of oral microbiota, therefore, in combination with novel drugs and delivery approaches serves as promising interventions and opportunities [188]. The application of ecological principles can help us understand how the tight interplay of the oral microbiota and the host dictates health or disease. We encourage advancing research directed toward developing ways or strategies to shift from traditional treatment to preventive and personalized dentistry.

6. Future directions for Philippine-based research and policy: oral microbiome and dental diseases in focus

The oral cavity is inhabited by hundreds of bacterial species that play vital roles in maintaining oral health or in shifting to a diseased state such as dental caries. The observed bacterial profile of the Filipinos compared with other populations may be brought about by the difference in their diet or oral hygiene practices. However, the possibility of this correlation has not been covered in a previous study on the Filipino oral microbiome [73]. Other factors influencing the shifts in the oral microbial diversity from a healthy to a diseased state may also be the focus of future studies.

The continued advancement of research and the resulting robust data on the oral microbiome is expected to lead to evidence-informed dentistry. The link of oral health diseases to systemic conditions have been established. Effective preventive measures, accurate diagnosis, sound treatment and the maintenance of good oral health will be expected outcomes when updated information on the oral microbiome are utilized optimally and may also lead to a decrease of the global burden of non-communicable diseases such as heart disease and diabetes mellitus. This strengthens the call for enhanced research on the Filipino oral microbiome and to shift the perspective that knowledge of the oral microbiome transcends health of the oral cavity but the general well-being of the individual and the populace.

Addressing the 87.4% dental caries and 48.3% periodontal disease prevalence [189] among Filipinos will not only require a responsive oral health care system but behavioral changes for Filipinos to prioritize oral health. The Lifecycle Approach has been laid out by the Department of Health in the delivery of the Basic Package of Oral Health Care [190]. Preventive Services must be done to provide specific protection from the occurrence of dental caries and other dental diseases, and this is initiated by the careful checking of the oral cavity.

Kits to test salivary pH levels are currently available. With its results analyzed with dietary patterns and oral hygiene habits, an individual's caries risk can be assessed. Minimum clinical intervention are done when appropriate preventive measures are adopted. Diagnostic tests to assess the oral microbiome were not specified in the DOH guidelines but utilization of these test kits, when available, can

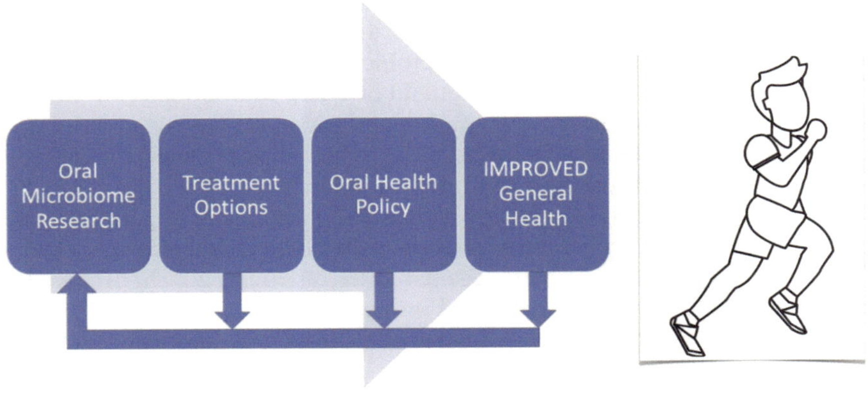

Figure 2.
Proposed framework directing possible future directions in Philippine-based research and policy focusing on Oral microbiome and dental caries.

aid in the development of individualized preventive programs. It should be noted that though the dental public health implications of diagnostic tests may be limited at the moment, its genomic value may be of promise. The high prevalence of oral diseases in the Philippines necessitates that unmet clinical needs be provided with proper preventive and promotive interventions. The development of a Filipino Oral Microbiome Database may support the advancement of effective oral health treatment options which could support responsive oral health policies in establishing oral health programs for Filipinos.

Figure 2 describes our proposed framework directing possible future directions in Philippine-based Research and Policy Focusing on Oral Microbiome and Dental Caries. It should be emphasized that monitoring and evaluation must be included in all stages. The process must be dynamic enough to allow for review. All stakeholders must be open to conducting new research when the desired outcomes are not being realized. With the enactment of the Universal Health Care (UHC) Act in 2018, the State is mandated to provide a comprehensive and integrated health care model to all Filipinos that include cost-effective promotive and preventive services. The translational data from oral microbiome researches can be referred for Health Technology Assessment to be reviewed for inclusion in the oral health care packages under the UHC.

Author details

Marilen P. Balolong[1*] and Michael Antonio F. Mendoza[2]

1 Department of Biology, College of Arts and Sciences, University of the Philippines Manila, Philippines

2 Department of Community Dentistry, College of Dentistry, University of the Philippines Manila, Philippines

*Address all correspondence to: mpbalolong2020@gmail.com and mpbalolong@up.edu.ph

References

[1] Sender R, Fuchs S, Milo R. Revised estimates for the number of human and bacteria cells in the body. PLoS Biology. 2016;**14**(8):e1002533

[2] Relman DA. The human microbiome: Ecosystem resilience and health. Nutrition Reviews. 2012;**70**(Suppl 1): S2-S9

[3] Yamashita Y, Takeshita T. The oral microbiome and human health. Journal of Oral Science. 2017;**59**:201-206

[4] Patil S, Rao RS, Amrutha N, Sanketh DS. Oral microbial flora in health. World J Dent. 2013;**4**:262-266

[5] Dewhirst FE, Chen T, Izard J, Paster BJ, Tanner AC, Yu WH, et al. The human oral microbiome. Journal of Bacteriology. 2010;**192**:5002-5017

[6] He J, Li Y, Cao Y, Xue J, Zhou X. The oral microbiome diversity and its relation to human diseases. Folia Microbiologica. 2015;**60**(1):69-80

[7] Zhao H, Chu M, Huang Z, Yang X, Ran S, Hu B, et al. Variations in oral microbiota associated with oral cancer. Sci Rep-Uk. 2017;**7**(1):11773

[8] Caselli E, Fabbri C, D'Accolti M, Soffritti BC, Mazzacane S, Franchi M. Defining the oral microbiome by whole-genome sequencing and resistome analysis: The complexity of the healthy picure. BMC Microbiology. 2020;**20**:120

[9] Deo PN, Deshmukh R. Oral microbiome: Unveiling the fundamentals. J Oral Maxillofac Pathol. 2019;**23**(1):122-128

[10] Verma D, Garg PK, Dubey AK. Insights into the human oral microbiome. Archives of Microbiology. 2018;**200**:525-540

[11] Krishnan K, Chen T, Paster BJ. A practical guide to the oral microbiome and its relation to health and disease. Oral Diseases. 2017;**23**(3):276-286

[12] Backhed F, Fraser CM, Ringel Y, Sanders ME, Sartor RB, Sherman PM, et al. Defining a healthy human gut microbiome: Current concepts, future directions, and clinical applications. Cell Host & Microbe. 2012;**12**(5):611-622

[13] Wade WG. The oral microbiome in health and disease. Pharmacological Research. 2013;**69**(1):137-143

[14] Aas JA, Paster BJ, Stokes LN, Olsen I, Dewhirst FE. Defining the normal bacterial flora of the oral cavity. Journal of Clinical Microbiology. 2005;**43**:5721-5732

[15] Aas JA, Griffen AL, Dardis SR, Lee AM, Olsen I, Dewhirst FE, et al. Bacteria of dental caries in primary and permanent teeth in children and young adults. Journal of Clinical Microbiology. 2008;**46**:1407-1417

[16] Paster BJ, Boches SK, Galvin JL, Ericson RE, Lau CN, Levanos VA, et al. Bacterial diversity in human subgingival plaque. Journal of Bacteriology. 2001; **183**:3770-3783

[17] Paster BJ, Olsen I, Aas JA, Dewhirst FE. The breadth of bacterial diversity in the human periodontal pocket and other oral sites. Periodontology 2000. 2006; **42**:80-87

[18] Batabyal B, Chakraborty S, Biswas S. Role of oral microflora in human population: A brief review. Int J Pharm Life Sci. 2012;**3**:2220-2227

[19] Marsh PD. Role of the oral microflora in health. Microbiol Ecol Health Dis. 2009;**12**:130-137

[20] Sampiao-Maia B, Monteiro-Silva F. Acquisition and maturation of oral

microbiome throughout childhood: An update. Dent Res J (Isfahan). 2014;**11**: 291-301

[21] Baker JL, Edlund A. Exploiting the Oral microbiome to prevent tooth decay: Has evolution already provided the best tools? Frontiers in Microbiology. 2019;**9**:3323

[22] Adler CJ, Dobney K, Weyrich LS, Kaidonis J, Walker AW, Haak W, et al. Sequencing ancient calcified dental plaque shows changes in oral microbiota with dietary shifts of the Neolithic and industrial revolutions. Nature Genetics. 2013;**45**:450-455

[23] Pitts NB, Zero DT, Marsh PD, Ekstrand K, Weintraub JA, Ramos-Gomez F, et al. Dental caries. Nature Reviews. Disease Primers. 2017;**3**:17030

[24] Human Microbiome Project C. A framework for human microbiome research. Nature. 2012; 486:215–21. [PubMed: 22699610

[25] Human Microbiome Project C. Structure, function and diversity of the healthy human microbiome. Nature. 2012c; 486:207–14. [PubMed: 22699609]

[26] Segata N, Haake SK, Mannon P, Lemon KP, Waldron L, Gevers D, et al. Composition of the adult digestive tract bacterial microbiome based on seven mouth surfaces, tonsils, throat and stool samples. Genome Biology. 2012;**13**:R42

[27] Zaura E, Keijser BJF, Huse SM, Crielaard W. Defining the healthy "core microbiome" of oral microbial communities. BMC Microbiology. 2009; **9**:259

[28] Gross EL, Leys EJ, Gasparovich SR, Firestone ND, Schwartzbaum JA, Janies DA, et al. Bacterial 16S sequence analysis of severe caries in young permanent teeth. Journal of Clinical Microbiology. 2010;**48**(11):4121-4128

[29] Nyvad B, Crielaard W, Mira A, Takahashi N, Beighton D. Dental caries from a molecular microbiological perspective. Caries Research. 2013;**47**: 89-102

[30] Hurley E, Mullins D, Barrett MP, O'Shea CA, Kinirons M, Anthony Ryan C, et al. The microbiota of the mother at birth and its influence on the emerging infant oral microbiota from birth to 1 year of age: A cohort study. Journal of Oral Microbiology. 2019;**11**:1

[31] Zhang Y, Wang X, Li H, Ni C, Du Z, and Yan F. 2018. Human oral microbiota and its modulation for oral health. *Biomed Pharmacother (Biomedecine pharmacotherapie)* 99:883–893.

[32] Krom BP, Kidwai S, Ten Cate JM. Candida and other fungal species: Forgotten players of healthy oral microbiota. Journal of Dental Research. 2014;**93**(5):445-451

[33] Dridi B, Raoult D, Drancourt M. Archaea as emerging organisms in complex human microbiomes. Anaerobe. 2011;**17**(2):56-63

[34] Nguyen-Hieu T, Khelaifia S, Aboudharam G, Drancourt M. Methanogenic archaea in subgingival sites: A review. APMIS. 2013;**121**(6): 467-477

[35] Kumaraswamy KL, Vidhya M. Human papilloma virus and oral infections: An update. Journal of Cancer Research and Therapeutics. 2011;**7**(2): 120-127

[36] Reznik DA. Oral manifestations of HIV disease. Top HIV Med. 2006;**13**: 143-148

[37] Lazarevic V, Whiteson K, Gaïa N, Gizard Y, Hernandez D, Farinelli L, et al. Analysis of the salivary microbiome using culture-independent techniques. Journal of Clinical Bioinformatics. 2012; **2**(1):4

[38] Abusleme L, Dupuy AK, Dutzan N, Silva N, Burleson JA, Strausbaugh LD, et al. The subgingival microbiome in health and periodontitis and its relationship with community biomass and inflammation. The ISME Journal. 2013;7(5):1016-1025

[39] Fan X, Alekseyenko AV, Wu J, Peters BA, Jacobs EJ, Gapstur SM, et al. Human oral microbiome and prospective risk for pancreatic cancer: A population-based nested case-control study. Gut. 2018;**67**:120-127

[40] Kerr AR. The oral microbiome and cancer. Journal of Dental Hygiene. 2015; **89**(Suppl 1):20-23

[41] Beck JD, Offenbacher S. Systemic effects of periodontitis: Epidemiology of periodontal disease and cardiovascular disease. Journal of Periodontology. 2005;**76**(11 Suppl):2089-2100

[42] Ley RE, Turnbaugh PJ, Klein S, Gordon JI. Microbial ecology: Human gut microbes associated with obesity. Nature. 2006;**444**(7122):1022-1023

[43] Turnbaugh, P. J. et al. The effect of diet on the human gut microbiome: a metagenomic analysis in humanized gnotobiotic mice. Science Translational Medicine 1, 6ra14–6ra14 (2009).

[44] Leishman SJ, Do HL, Ford PJ. Cardiovascular disease and the role of oral bacteria. Journal of Oral Microbiology. 2010. DOI: 10.3402/jom.v2i0.5781

[45] Demmer RT, Jacobs DR Jr, Singh R, Zuk A, Rosenbaum M, Papapanou PN, and Desvarieux M. 2015. Periodontal bacteria and prediabetes prevalence in origins: the oral infections, glucose intolerance, and insulin resistance study. *J Dent Res.*94:201S – 211S.

[46] Docktor MJ, Paster BJ, Abramowicz S, Ingram J, Wang YE, Correll M, et al. Alterations in diversity of the oral microbiome in pediatric inflammatory bowel disease. Inflammatory Bowel Diseases. 2012;**18**:935-942

[47] Farrell JJ, Zhang L, Zhou H, Chia D, Elashoff D, Akin D, et al. Variations of oral microbiota are associated with pancreatic diseases including pancreatic cancer. Gut. 2012;**61**:582-588

[48] Ahn J, Sinha R, Pei Z, Dominianni C, Wu J, Shi J, et al. Human gut microbiome and risk for colorectal cancer. Journal of the National Cancer Institute. 2013;**105**(24):1907-1911

[49] Foster JA, McVey Neufeld KA. Gut-brain axis: How the microbiome influences anxiety and depression. Trends in Neurosciences. 2013;**36**(5): 305-312

[50] Acharya A, Chan Y, Kheur S, Jin LJ, Watt RM, Mattheos N. Salivary microbiome in non-oral disease: A summary of evidence and commentary. Archives of Oral Biology. 2017;**83**: 169-173

[51] Gibbons RJ. Bacteriology of dental caries. Journal of Dental Research. 1964; **43**(6):1021-1028

[52] Loesche WJ, Rowan J, Straffon LH, Loos PJ. Association of Streptococcus mutans with dental decay. Infection and Immunity. 1975;**11**(6):1252-1260

[53] Loesche WJ, Straffon LH. Longitudinal investigation of the role of Streptococcus mutans in human fissure decay. Infection and Immunity. 1979;**26** (2):498-507

[54] Harper DS, Loesche WJ. Growth and tolerance of human dental plaque bacteria. Archives of Oral Biology. 1984; **29**(10):843-848

[55] Loesche WJ. Role of Streptococcus mutans in human dental decay. Microbiological Reviews. 1986;**50**(4): 353-380

[56] Bradshaw DJ, McKee AS, Marsh PD. The use of defined inocula stored in liquid nitrogen for mixed-culture chemostat studies. J Microbiol Meth. 1989;**9**:123-128

[57] Kneist S, Scharff S, de Soet JJ, van Loveren C, Stosser L. Bacteriocin production by human strains of mutans and oral streptococci. Caries Res. 2000; **34**:308

[58] Bradshaw DJ, Homer KA, Marsh PD, Beighton D. Metabolic cooperation in oral microbial communities during growth on mucin. Microbiology. 1994; **140**(Pt 12):3407-3412

[59] Mantzourani M, Gilbert SC, Sulong HNH, Sheehy EC, Tank S, Fenlon M, et al. The isolation of bifidobacteria from occlusal carious lesions in children and adults. Caries Research. 2009;**43**: 308-313

[60] Vartoukian SR, Palmer RM, Wade WG. Cultivation of a Synergistetes strain representing a previously uncultivated lineage. Environmental Microbiology. 2010;**12**:916-928

[61] Zawadzki PJ, Perkowski K, Padzik M, Mierzwińska-Nastalska E, Szaflik JP, Conn DB, et al. Examination of oral microbiota diversity in adults and older adults as an approach to prevent spread of risk factors for human infections. *BioMed Research International*. 2017; **2017**:8106491

[62] Hooper SJ, Crean SJ, Lewis MAO, Spratt DA, Wade WG, Wilson MJ. Viable bacteria present within oral squamous cell carcinoma tissue. Journal of Clinical Microbiology. 2006;**44**(5): 1719-1725

[63] Dalwai F, Spratt DA, Pratten J. Use of quantitative PCR and culture methods to characterize ecological flux in bacterial biofilms. Journal of Clinical Microbiology. 2007;**45**(9):3073-3076

[64] Piwat S, Teanpaisan R, Thitasomakul S, Thearmontree A, Dahlén G. Lactobacillus species and genotypes associated wih dental caries in Thai preschool children. Molecular Oral Microbiology. 2010;**25**(2):157-164

[65] Bik EM, Long CD, Armitage GC, Loomer P, Emerson J, Mongodin EF, et al. Bacterial diversity in the oral cavity of 10 healthy individuals. *The ISME* Journal. 2010;**4**:962-974

[66] Xie G, Chain PSG, Lo CC, Liu KL, Gans J, Merritt J, et al. Community and gene composition of a human dental plaque microbiota obtained by metagenomic sequencing. Molecular Oral Microbiology. 2010;**25**:391-405

[67] Yang R, Argimon S, Li Y, Gu H, Zhou X, Caufield PW. Determining the genetic diversity of lactobacilli from the oral cavity. Journal of Microbiological Methods. 2010;**82**(2):163-169

[68] ACR T, Kent RL Jr, Lif Holgerson P, Hughes CV, Loo CY, Kanasi E, et al. Microbiota of severe early childhood caries before and after therapy. Journal of Dental Research. 2011;**90**(11): 1298-1305

[69] Alcaraz LD, Belda-Ferre P, Cabrera-Rubio R, Romero H, Simón-Soro Á, Pignatelli M, et al. Identifying healthy oral microbiome through metagenomics. Clinical Microbiology and Infection. 2012;**18**(4):54-57

[70] Belda-Ferre P, Alcaraz LD, Cabrera-Rubio R, Romero H, Simon-Soro A, Pignatelli M, et al. The oral metagenome in health and disease. The ISME Journal. 2012;**6**:46-56

[71] Kawamura Y, Kamiya Y. Metagenomic analysis permit- ting identification of the minority bacterial populations in the oral microbiota. J. Oral Biosci. 2012;**54**:132-137

[72] Pushalkar S, Ji X, Li Y, Estilo C, Yegnanarayana R, Singh B, et al.

Comparison of oral microbiota in tumor and non-tumor tissues of patients with oral squamous cell carcinoma. BMC Microbiology. 2012;**12**:144

[73] Reyes CPA, Dalmacio LMM. Bacterial diversity in the saliva and plaque of caries free and caries-active Filipino adults. Philippine Journal of Science. 2012;**141** (2):217-227

[74] Yang F, Zeng X, Ning K, Liu KL, Wang W, Chen J, et al. Saliva microbiomes distinguish caries-active from healthy human populations. The ISME Journal. 2012;**6**(1):1-10

[75] Benitez-Paez A, Belda-Ferre P, Simon-Soro A, Mira A. Microbiota diversity and gene expression dynamics in human oral biofilms. BMC Genomics. 2014;**15**:311

[76] Mason MR, Preshaw PM, Nagaraja HN, Dabdoub SM, Rahman A, Kumar PS. He subgingival microbiome of clinically healthy current and never smokers. The ISME Journal. 2015;**9**(10): 268-272

[77] Schmidt BL, Kuczynski J, Bhattacharya A, Huey B, Corby PM, Queiroz ELS, et al. Changes in abundance or oral microbiota associated with oral cancer. PLoS One. 2014;**9**(8): e106297

[78] Banas JA, Zhu M, Dawson DV, Cao H, Levy SM. PCR-based identification of oral streptococcal species. Int J Dent. 2016;**2016**:3465163

[79] Dame-Teixeira N, Parolo CCF, Maltz M, Tugnait A, Devine D, and Do T. 2016. Actinomyces spp. gene expression in root canal lesions. *J Oral Microbiol* 8:10.3402.

[80] Fourie NH, Wang D, Abey SK, Sherwin LB, Joseph PV, Rahim-Williams B, Ferguson EG, and Henderson WA. The microbiome of the oral mucosa in irritable bowel syndrome. Gut Microbes. 2016;**7**:286-301

[81] Al-hebshi NN, Nasher AT, Maryoud MY, Homeida HE, Chen T, Idris AM, et al. Inflammatory bacteriome featuring *Fusobacterium nucleatum* and *Pseudomonas aeruginosa* identified in association with oral squamous cell carcinoma. Scientific Reports. 2017;7: 1834

[82] Ganesan SM, Joshi V, Fellows M, Dabdoub SM, Nagaraja HN. A tale of two risks: Smoking diabetes and the subgingival microbiome. The ISME Journal. 2017;**11**:2075-2089

[83] Lassalle F, Spagnoletti M, Fumagalli M, Shaw L, Dyble M, Walker C, et al. Oral microbiomes from hunter-gatherers and traditional farmers reveal shifts in commensal balance and pathogen load linked to diet. Mol Ecol. 2018 Jan;**27**(1):182-195. DOI: 10.1111/mec.14435

[84] Mashima I, Theodorea CF, Thaweboon B, Thaweboon S, Scannapieco FA, Nakazawa F. Exploring the salivary microbiome of children stratified by the oral hygiene index. PLoS One. 2017;**12**(9):e0185274

[85] Si J, Lee C, Ko G. Oral microbiota: Microbial biomarkers of metabolic syndrome independent of host genetic factors. Frontiers in Cellular and Infection Microbiology. 2017;7:516

[86] Chen WP, Chang SH, Tang CY, Liou ML, Tsai SJJ, Lin YL. Composition analysis and feature selection of the oral microbiota associated with periodontal disease. BioMed Research International. 2018;**2018**:3130607

[87] Thurnheer T, Belibasakis GN. Streptococus oralis maintains homeostasis in oral biofilms by antagonizing the cariogenic pathogen Streptococus mutans. Molecular Oral Microbiology. 2018;**33**(3):234-239

[88] Carda-Diéguez M, Bravo-González LA, Morata IM, Vicente A, Mira A. High-throughput DNA sequencing of microbiota at interproximal sites. Journal of Oral Microbiology. 2020;**12** (1):1687397

[89] Jiang Q, Liu J, Chen L, Gan N, Yang D. The Oral Microbiome in the Elderly With Dental Caries and Health. *Front Cell Infect Microbiol*. 2019;8:442. Published 2019 Jan 4. doi:10.3389/fcimb.2018.00442

[90] Raju SC, Lagström S, Ellonen P, de Vos WM, Eriksson JG, Weiderpass E, et al. Gender-specific associations between saliva microbiota and body size. Frontiers in Microbiology. 2019;**10**:767

[91] Thurnheer T, Karygianni L, Flury M, and Belibasakis GN. 2019. Fusobacterium species and subspecies differentially affect the composition and architecture of supra- and subgingival biofilms models. *Front Microbiol* doi.org/10.3389/fmicb.2019.01716

[92] Burcham ZM, Garneau NL, Comstock SS, Tucker RM, Knight R, Metcalf JL and Genetics of Taste Lab Citizen Scientists. 2020. Patterns of Oral microbiota diversity in adults and children: A crowdsourced population study. Scientific Reports 10:2133.

[93] Kori J, Saleem F, Ullah S, Azim K. Characterization of Oral bacteriome dysbiosis in type 2 diabetic patients. In: medRxiv. 2020

[94] Handelsman J. Metagenomics: Application of genomics to uncultured microorganisms. Microbiology and Molecular Biology Reviews. 2002;**68**: 669-685

[95] Sizova M, Hohmann T, Hazen A, Paser BJ, Halem SR, Murphy CM, et al. New approaches for isolation of previously uncultivated oral bacteria. Applied and Environmental Microbiology. 2012;**78**:194-203

[96] Asikainen S, Karched M, Rogers A. Molecular Techniques in Oral Microbial Taxonomy Identifications and Typing. *Norfolk, UK*: *Caister Academic Press*; 2008

[97] Zaura E. Next-generation sequencing approaches to understanding the oral microbiome. Advances in Dental Research. 2012;**24**: 81-85

[98] Soro V, Dutton LC, Sprague SV, Nobbs AH, Ireland AJ, Sandy JR, et al. Axenic culture of a can- didate division TM7 bacterium from the human oral cavity and biofilm interactions with other oral bacteria. Applied and Environmental Microbiology. 2014;**80**: 6480-6489

[99] Wade WG. Unculturable bacteria—The uncharacterized organisms that cause oral infections. Journal of the Royal Society of Medicine. 2002;**95**: 81-83

[100] Jenkinson HF. Beyond the oral microbiome. Environmental Microbiology. 2011;**13**:3077-3087

[101] Siqueira JF Jr, Rôças IN. As-yet-uncultivated oral bacteria: Breadth and association with oral and extra-oral diseases. Journal of Oral Microbiology. 2013;**5**:1-14

[102] Benn A, Heng N, Broadbent JM, Thomson WM. 2018. Studying the human oral microbiome: Challenges and the evolution of solutions. Australian Dental Journal. *2018*;**63**:14-24

[103] Anderson IC, Cairney JW. Diversity and ecology of soil fungal communities: Increased understanding through the application of molecular techniques. Environmental Microbiology. 2004;**6**:769-779

[104] Nishigaki K, Naimuddin M, Hamano K. Genome profiling: A realistic solution for genotype-based

identification of species. Journal of Biochemistry. 2000;**128**:107-112

[105] Socransky SS, Smith C, Martin L, Paster BJ, Dewhirst FE, Levin AE. "Checkerboard" DNA-DNA hybridization. BioTechniques. 1994;**17**: 788-792

[106] Schena M, Shalon D, Davis RW, and Brown PO. 1995. Quantitative monitoring of gene expression patterns with a complementary DNA microarray. *Science*270:467–470.

[107] Chung SK. Oral metagenomic analysis techniques. J Dent Hyg Sci. 2019;**19**(2):86-95

[108] Chen K, Neimark H, Rumore P, Steinman CR. Broad-range DNA probes for detecting and amplifying eubacterial nucleic acids. FEMS Microbiology Letters. 1989;**57**:19-24

[109] Relman DA. The search for unrecognized pathogens. Science. 1999; **284**:1308-1310

[110] Yang B, Wang Y, Qian PY. Sensitivity and correlation of hypervariable regions in 16S rRNA genes in phylogenetic analysis. BMC Bioinformatics. 2016;**17**:135

[111] Chakravorty S, Helb D, Burday M, Connell N, Alland D. A detailed analysis of 16S ribosomal RNA gene segments for the diagnosis of pathogenic bacteria. Journal of Microbiological Methods. 2007;**69**:330-339

[112] Kumar PS, Brooker MR, Dowd SE, Camerlengo T. Target region selection is a critical determinant of community fingerprints generated by 16S pyrosequencing. PLoS One. 2011;**6**: e20956

[113] Kawamura Y, Fukunaga H, Hirose K, Ezaki T. Basic study of the LCR-MTB system. Clin Microbiol. 1998;**25**:873-874

[114] Kuwamura Y, Kamiya Y. Metagenomic analysis permitting identification of the minority bacterial populations in the oral microbiota. Journal of Oral Biosciences. 2012;**54**(3): 132-137

[115] Avila M, Ojcius DM, Yilmaz O. The oral microbiota: Living with a permanent guest. DNA and Cell Biology. 2009;**28**(8):405-411

[116] Elahi E, Ronaghi M. Pyrosequencing: A tool for DNA sequencing analysis. Methods in Molecular Biology. 2004;**255**:211-219

[117] Ames NJ, Ranucci A, Moriyama B, Wallen GR. The human microbiome and understanding the 16S rRNA gene in translational nursing science. Nursing Research. 2017;**66**(2):184-197

[118] Hasan NA, Young BA, Minard-Smith AT, Saeed K, Li H, Heizer EM, et al. Microbial community profiling of human saliva using shotgun metagenomic sequencing. PLoS One. 2014;**9**(5):e97699

[119] Yu G, Phillips S, Gail MH, Goedert JJ, Humphrys M, Ravel J, et al. Evaluation of buccal cell samples for studies of oral microbiota. Cancer Epidemiology, Biomarkers & Prevention. 2017;**26**:249-253

[120] Clemente JC, Pehrsson EC, Blaser MJ, Sandhu K, Gao Z, Wang B, Magris M, Hidalgo G, Contreras M, Noya-Alarcon O, Lander O, McDonald J, Cox M, Walter J, Oh PL, Ruiz JF, Rodriguez S, Shen N, Song SJ, Metcalf J, Knight R, Dantas G, Dominguez-Bello MG. 2015. The microbiome of uncontacted Amerindians. Sci Adv. 2015;1:e1500183.

[121] Lim MY, Cho Y, Rho M. Diverse distribution of Resistomes in the human and environmental microbiomes. Current Genomics. 2018;**19**(8):701-711

[122] Choi Y-H, Kosaka T, Ojima M, Sekini S, Kokubo Y, Watanabe M, et al.

Relationship between the burden of major periodontal bacteria and serum lipid profile in a cross-sectional Japanese study. BMC Oral Health. 2018;**18**(1):77

[123] Topcuoglu N, Kulekci G. 16S rRNA based microarray analysis of ten periodontal bacteria in patients with different forms of periodontitis. Anaerobe, Volume 35. Part A. 2015; **2015**:35-40

[124] Zheng H, Xu L, Wang Z, Li L, Zhang J, Zhang Q, et al. Subgingival microbiome in patients with healthy and ailing dental implants. Sci Rep. 2015 Jun 16;**5**:10948

[125] Hu X, Zhang Q, Hua H, Chen F. Changes in the salivary microbiota of oral leukoplakia and oral cancer. Oral Oncol. 2016;**56**:6-8

[126] Amer A, Galvin S, Healy CM, Moran GP. The microbiome of potentially malignant oral leukoplakia exhibits enrichment for Fusobacterium, Leptotrichia, Campylobacter, and Rothia species. Front Microbiol. 2017;**8**: 2391-2400

[127] Wang Y, Zhang J, Chen X, et al. Profiling of oral microbiota in early childhood caries using single-molecule real-time sequencing. Front Microbiol. 2017;**8**:2244

[128] Agnello M, Cen L, Tran NC, Shi W, Mclean JS, He X. Arginine improves pH homeostasis via metabolism and microbiome modulation. J. Dent. Res. 2017;**96**:924-930

[129] Said HS, Suda W, Nakagome S, Chinen H, Oshima K, Kim S, Kimura R, Iraha A, Ishida H, Fujita J, Mano S, Morita H, Dohi T. Oota H, and Hattori M. 2014. Dysbiosis of salivary microbiota in inflammatory bowel disease and its association with oral immunological biomarkers. DNA Research 21:15–25.

[130] Mager DL, Haffajee AD, Devlin PM, Norris CM, Posner MR, Goodson JM. The salivary microbiota as a diagnostic indicator of oral cancer: a descriptive, non-randomized study of cancer-free and oral squamous cell carcinoma subjects. J Transl Med. 2005;**3**:27

[131] Mager DL, Haffajee AD, Devlin PM, Norris CM, Posner MR, Goodson JM. The salivary microbiota as a diagnostic indicator of oral cancer: a descriptive, non-randomized study of cancer-free and oral squamous cell carcinoma subjects. J Transl Med. 2005;**3**:27

[132] Pushalkar S, Mane SP, Ji X, et al. Microbial Diversity in Saliva of Oral Squamous Cell carcinoma. FEMS Immunol Med Microbiol. 2011;**61**(3): 269-277

[133] Al-Hebshi NN, Nasher AT, Maryoud MY, et al. Inflammatory bacteriome featuring Fusobacetrium nucleatum and pseudomonas aeruginosa identified in association with oral squamous cell carcinoma. Sci Rep. 2017; **7**(1):1834

[134] Lee WH, Chen H-M, Yang S-F, Liang C, Peng C-Y, Lin F-M, et al. Bacterial alterations in salivary microbiota and their association in oral cancer. Sci. Rep. 2017;**7**

[135] Torres PJ, Fletcher EM, Gibbons SM, Bouvet M, Doran KS, Kelley ST. Characterization of the salivary microbiome in patients with pancreatic cancer. PerrJ 2015; 3e1373

[136] Fan X, Alekseyenko AV, Wu J, Peters BA, Jacobs EJ, Gapstur SM, et al. Human oral microbiome and prospective risk for pancre- atic cancer: a population-based nested case-control study. Gut. 2016;**67**(1):120-127

[137] Olson SH, Satagopan J, Xu Y, et al. The oral microbiota in patients with

pancreatic cancer, patients with IPMNs and controls: a pilot study. Cancer Causes Control. 2017;**28**(9):959-969

[138] Lu H, Ren Z, Li A. Tongue coating microbiome data distinguish patients with pancreatic head cancer from health controls. Journal of Oral Microbiology. 2019;**11**(1):1563409

[139] Katz J, Onate MD, Pauley KM, Bhattacharyya I, Cha S. Presence of Porphyromonas gingivalis in gingival squamous cell carcinoma. Int J Oral Sci. 2011;**3**(4):209-215

[140] Guerrero-Preston R, White JR, Godoy-Vitorino F, et al. High-resolution microbiome profiling uncovers Fusobacterium nucleatum, lactobacillus gasseri/johnsonii and Lactobacillus vaginalis associated to oral and oropharyngeal cancer in saliva from HPV-positive and HPOV negative patients treated with surgery and chemo-radiation. Oncotarget. 2017;**8** (67):110931-110948

[141] Decsi G, Soki J, Pap B, Dobra G, Harmati M, Kormondi S, et al. Chicken or the egg: Microbial alterations in biopsy samples of patients with oral potentially malignant disorders. Pathol Oncol Res. 2018. [PMID: 30054809]

[142] Scalas D, Roana J, Boffano P, et al. Bacteriological findings in radicuylar cyst and keratocystic odontogenic tumuor fludis from asymptomatic patients. Arch Oral Biol. 2013;**58**(11): 1578-1583

[143] Flemer B, Lynch DB, Brown JM, et al. Tumour-associated and non-tumour-associated microbiota in colorectal cancer. Gut. 2017;**66**(4): 633-643

[144] Peters BA, Wu J, Pei Z, Yang L, Purdue MP, Freedman ND, et al. Oral Microbiome composition reflects prospective risk for esophageal cancers. Cancer Res. 2017;**77**(23):6777-6787

[145] Chen, H., Liu, Y., Zhang, M., Wang, G., Qi, Z., Bridgewater, L., ... Pang, X. (2015). A Filifactor alocis-centered co-occurrence group associates with periodontitis across different oral habitats. Scientific Reports, 5.

[146] Wu J, Xu S, Xiang C, et al. Tongue Coating Microbiota Community and Risk Effect on Gastric Cancer. J Cancer. 2018;**9**(21):4039-4048

[147] Mukherjee PK, Wang H, Retuerto M, et al. Bacteriome and mycobiome associatoons in oral tongue cancer. Oncotarget. 2017;**8**(57):97273-97289

[148] Kamer AR, Craig RG, Pirraglia E, Dasanayake AP, Norman RG, Boylan RJ, et al. TNF-alpha and antibodies to periodontal bacteria discriminate between Alzheimer's disease patients and normal subjects. J Neuroimmunol. 2009;**216**:92-97

[149] Kamer AR, Craig RG, Pirraglia E, Dasanayake AP, Norman RG, Boylan RJ, et al. TNF-alpha and antibodies to periodontal bacteria discriminate between Alzheimer's disease patients and normal subjects. J Neuroimmunol. 2009;**216**:92-97

[150] Casarin RC, Barbagallo A, Meulman T, Santos VR, Sallum EA, Nociti FH, et al. Subgingival biodiversity in subjects with uncontrolled type-2 diabetes and chronic periodontitis. J Periodontal Res. 2013;**48**(1):30-36

[151] Madianos PN, Bobetsis YA, Offenbacher S. Adverse pregnancy outcomes (APOs) and periodontal disease: Patho- genic mechanisms. Journal of Clinical Periodontology. 2013; **40**(14):S170-S180

[152] Han YW, Fardini Y, Chen C, Iacampo KG, Peraino VA, Shamonki JM, et al. Term stillbirth caused by oral Fusobacterium nucleatum. Obstetrics and Gynecology. 2010;**115**:442-445

[153] Zhang X, Zhang D, Jia H, Feng Q, Wang D, Liang D, et al. The oral and gut microbiomes are perturbed in rheumatoid arthritis and partly normalized after treatment. Nature Medicine. 2015;**21**(8):895-905

[154] Dang AT, Cotton S, Sankaran-Walters S, Li CS, Lee CY, Dandekar S, et al. Evidence of an increased pathogenic footprint in the lingual micro- biome of untreated HIV infected patients. BMC Microbiol. 2012;**12**:153

[155] Koren O, Spor A, Felin J, Fak F, Stombaugh J, Tremaroli V, et al. Human oral, gut, and plaque mi- crobiota in patients with atherosclerosis. Proc. Natl. Acad. Sci. U. S. A. 2011;**108**(Suppl. 1): 4592-4598

[156] Rôças IN, Alves FRF, Rachid CTCC, Lima KC, Assunção IV, Gomes PN, Siqueira JFJr. 2016. Microbiome of deep dentinal caries lesions in teeth with symptomatic irreversible pulpitis. *PLoS One* 2016;11:e0154653.

[157] Takeshita T, Matsuo K, Furuta M, Shibata Y, Fukami K, Shimazaki Y, et al. Distinct composition of the oral indigenous microbiota in south Korean and Japanese adults. Scientific Reports. 2014;**4**:6990

[158] Zhou J, Jiang N, Wang S, Hu X, Jiao K, He X, et al. Exploration of human salivary microbiomes-insights into the novel characteristics of microbial community structure in caries and caries-free subjects. PLoS One. 2016;**11** (1):e0147039

[159] Han YW, Wang X. Mobile microbiome: Oral bacteria in extra-oral infections and inflammation. Journal of Dental Research. 2013;**92**:485-491

[160] Gao L, Xu T, Huang G, Jiang S, Gu Y, Chen F. Oral microbiomes: More and more importance in oral cavity and whole body. Protein & Cell. 2018;**9**(5): 488-500

[161] Huang X, Palmer SR, Ahn SJ, Richards VP, Williams ML, Nascimento MM, et al. A highly arginolytic streptococcus species that potently antagonizes Streptococcus mutans. Applied and Environmental Microbiology. 2016;**82**:2187-2201

[162] Curtis MA. Periodontal microbiology - the lid's off the box again. Journal of Dental Research. 2014; **93**:840-842

[163] Yakob M, Fuentes L, Wang MB, Abemayor E, Wong DTW. Salivary biomarkers for detection of oral squamous cell carcinoma: Current state and recent advances. Curr Oral Health Rep. 2014;**1**:133-141

[164] Marsh PD. In sickness and in health-what does the oral microbiome mean to us? An ecological perspective. Advances in Dental Research. 2018;**29** (1):60-65

[165] Johansson A, Claesson R, Höglund Åberg C, Haubek D, Lindholm M, Jasim S, et al. Genetic profiling of Aggregatibacter actinomycetemcomitans serotype B isolated from periodontitis patients living in Sweden. Pathogens. 2019; **8**(3):153

[166] Esberg A, Sheng N, Mårell L, Claesson R, Persson K, Borén T, et al. Streptococcus Mutans adhesin biotypes that match and predict individual caries development. EBio Med. 2017;**24**: 205-215

[167] Yamanaka W, Takeshita T, Shibata Y, Matsuo K, Eshima N, Yokoyama T, et al. Compositional stability of a salivary bacterial population against supragingival microbiota shift following periodontal therapy. PLoS One. 2012;**7** (8):e42806

[168] Nathan C. Antibiotics at the crossroads. Nature. 2004;**431**(7011): 899-902

[169] Ready D, Lancaster H, Qureshi F, Bedi R, Mullany P, Wilson M. Effect of amoxicillin use on oral microbiota in young children. Antimicrobial Agents and Chemotherapy. 2004;**48**(8):2883-2887

[170] Guarner F, Perdigon G, Corthier G, Salminen S, Koletzko B, Morelli L. Should yoghurt cultures be considered probiotic? The British Journal of Nutrition. 2005;**93**(6):783-786

[171] Teughels W, Loozen G, Quirynen M. Do probiotics offer opportunities to manipulate the periodontal oral microbiota? Journal of Clinical Periodontology. 2011;**38**:159-177

[172] Lingam L, Ramesh T, Lavanya R. Bacteria in oral health-probiotics and prebiotics a review. Int. J. Biol. Med. Res. 2011;**2**(4):1226-1233

[173] Meurman JH, Stamatova I. Probiotics: Contributions to oral health. Oral Diseases. 2007;**13**(5):443-451

[174] Busscher H, Mulder A, Van der Mei H. In vitro adhesion to enamel and in vivo colonization of tooth surfaces by lactobacilli from a bio–yoghurt. Caries Research. 1999;**33**(5):403-404

[175] Näse L, Hatakka K, Savilahti E, Saxelin M, Pönkä A, Poussa T, et al. Effect of of long–term consumption of a probiotic bacterium, lactobacillus rhamnosus GG, in milk on dental caries and caries risk in children. Caries Research. 2001;**35**(6):412-420

[176] Caglar E, Sandalli N, Twetman S, Kavaloglu S, Ergeneli S, Selvi S. Effect of yogurt with bifidobacterium DN-173 010 on salivary mutans streptococci and lactobacilli in young adults. Acta Odontologica Scandinavica. 2005;**63**(6):317-320

[177] Caglar E, Kavaloglu S, Cildir S, Ergeneli S, Sandalli N, Twetman S. Salivary mutans streptococci and lactobacilli levels after ingestion of the probiotic bacterium lactobacillus reuteri ATCC 55730 by straws or tablets. Acta Odontologica Scandinavica. 2006;**64**(5):314-318

[178] Cildir SK, Germec D, Sandalli N, Ozdemir FI, Arun T, Twetman S, et al. Reduction of salivary mutans streptococci in orthodontic patients during daily consumption of yoghurt containing probiotic bacteria. European Journal of Orthodontics. 2009;**31**(4):407-411

[179] Holz C, Alexander C, Balcke C, More M, Auinger A, Bauer M, et al. Lactobacillus paracasei DSMZ16671 reduces mutans streptococci: A short-term pilot study. Probiotics Antimicrob. Proteins. 2013;**5**:259-263

[180] Ohshima T, Kojima Y, Seneviratne CJ, Maeda N. Therapeutic application of synbiotics, a fusion of probiotics and prebiotics, and biogenics as a new concept for oral Candida infections: A mini review. *Front Microbiol* doi. 2016. DOI: 10.3389/fmicb.2016.00010

[181] Zarco MF, Vess TJ, Ginsburg GS. The oral microbiome in health and disease and the potential impact on personalized dental medicine. Oral Diseases. 2012;**18**(2):109-120

[182] Tagg JR, Dierksen KP. Bacterial replacement therapy: Adapting' germ warfare' to infection prevention. Trends in Biotechnology. 2003;**21**(5):217-223

[183] Ren Z et al. Dual-targeting approach degrades biofilm matrix and enhances bacterial killing. J. Dent. Res. 2019;**98**:322-330

[184] Paisano AF, Spira B, Cai S, Bombana AC. In vitro antimicrobial effect bacteriophages on human dentin infected with enterococcus faecalis ATCC 29212. *Oral Microbiol*. Immunol. 2004;**19**(5):327-330

[185] Benergossi J, Calixto G, Fonseca-Santos B, Aida KL, Negrini TC, Duque C, et al. Highlights in peptide nanoparticle carriers intended to oral diseases. Current Topics in Medicinal Chemistry. 2015;**15**(4):345-355

[186] Hearnden V, Sankar V, Hull K, Juras DV, Greenberg M, Kerr AR, et al. New developments and op- portunities in oral mucosal drug delivery for local and systemic disease. Advanced Drug Delivery Reviews. 2012;**64**(1):16-28

[187] Joshi D, Garg T, Goyal AK, Rath G. Advanced drug delivery approaches against periodontitis. Drug Delivery. 2016;**23**(2):363-377

[188] Rosier BT, Marsh PB, Mira A. Resilience of the Oral microbiota in health: Mechanisms that prevent dysbiosis. Journal of Dental Research. 2018;**97**(4):371-380

[189] Department of Health Philippines. National Monitoring & Evaluation Dental Survey (2011): Final Report. Philippines: Manila; 2013

[190] Department of Health Philippines. 2007. Administrative Order 2007–0007 Guidelines in Implementation of Oral Health Program for Public Health Services.

Chapter 5

The Application of Fluoride in Dental Caries

Haiyang Sun, Feng Luo and Qianbing Wan

Abstract

The most efficient way to prevent caries is by using fluoridated dental products. Fluoride can reduce enamel demineralization and promote enamel remineralization. In terms of prevention, the topical application of fluoride is accessible, which includes fluoride toothpaste, fluoride varnish, fluoride gel, and mouth rinse. Besides, the application of fluoride is systematical. In some countries, fluoride is added into water, salt, or milk. Fluoride is also used for the medical treatment of early dental caries. However, fluoride is a double-edged sword. Excessive fluoride intake will cause toxic reactions, and dental fluorosis is caused by a high intake of fluorides during tooth development.

Keywords: fluoride intake, caries prevention, fluorosis, fluoride application

1. Introduction

Fluorides are regarded as effective materials in the control of dental caries, which can both benefit the prevention and treatment.

Fluoride is widely distributed in nature and is present in all soils, water, plants, and animals [1]. Water-soluble fluoride in the soil is the most valuable for organisms. Because fluoride is not distributed in soil evenly, the concentration of fluoride in water is different in different areas. Plants generally contain a certain amount of fluoride, which is absorbed from the soil and water. Besides, plants can increase the content of fluoride by absorbing deposited fluoride on the leaves or absorbing the fluoride in the atmosphere directly. Fluoride in the atmosphere mainly comes from a volcanic eruption, industrial waste gas, and coal combustion [2, 3].

2. Fluoride: intake and mechanism

Most of the human fluoride comes from food and water [1]. The primary source of human fluoride is water. It is easy for the body to absorb fluoride from water. However, the amount of fluoride absorbed by the body from drinking water is directly controlled by the fluoride concentration and the amount of drinking water. The amount of drinking water depends on age, living habits, local temperature, and other factors. Adults drink about 2500–3000 ml of water per day. The second source of human fluoride is food. All foods, including plant or animal food, contain a certain amount of fluoride, but the content of fluoride among them is widely different. Plant food, such as grains, vegetables, fruits, and so on, often has significant differences in fluoride content due to different regions. The fluoride in the air is not the primary source of human fluoride. Unfortunately, under some special environmental conditions, air can be polluted by fluoride. In this way, the fluoride in the air can enter into the human body through the respiratory tract, causing fluorosis. In addition, there are other possible sources of fluoride. For example, some oral topical fluoride products have very high fluoride concentration. If they are used unproperly without the guidance of doctors, it may lead to an increase in fluoride intake. The total intake of fluoride is the sum of the intake of fluoride from the air, water, diet, and so on. It contains two meanings: one is the total adaptive intake, which refers to the physiological demand for preventing and maintaining normal biological functions of the body; the other is the total safe intake, which refers to the maximum amount that the body needs. When the body takes more chemicals than the safe intake for a long time, it will lead to chronic poisoning. It isn't very easy to unify the standard of appropriate intake and safe intake of fluorine, so we recommend the proper daily intake of fluorine is 0.05–0.07 mg [4].

At present, it is believed that the primary mechanism of fluoride to prevent caries is by reducing demineralization and promoting enamel remineralization. Besides, fluoride has effects on the microorganism.

Under normal conditions, the solubility of enamel in acid buffer varies according to the concentration of fluoride. When the concentration of fluoride reaches 0.05 mg/l, the solubility of enamel will be reduced. Fluorine can be combined with free hydroxyapatite (HA) to form fluorohydroxyapatite (FHA) in the saturated solution of hydroxyapatite, which can be redeposited in enamel. And this process is named remineralization. In contrast, when the hydroxyapatite in the solution is not saturated, fluorine can directly enter the crystal to form FHA or exchange with hydroxyl ion in enamel to form fluorapatite (FA). When the teeth are eroded by acid, the pH value decreases, and the teeth demineralize. At the same time, calcium fluoride dissolves and releases fluoride and calcium ions into saliva. When the calcium and phosphorus ions in saliva are saturated, they will make the minerals return to the teeth. If this process happens on the surface of the demineralized crystal, a new crystal surface will be formed.

In addition to preventing caries, dentists also use fluoride to treat dental caries [5]. The fluoride deposited on the surface of demineralized enamel can promote the remineralization of enamel and then play a role in treating dental caries. There are lots of fluorides reported to be used in the treatment of dental caries, mostly in the early stage of tooth decay, such as sodium fluoride (NaF) and silver diamine fluoride (SDF) [6]. A system review concluded that applying 38% SDF annually to older adults who had exposed root surfaces decreased the prevalence of new root carious lesions by at least 50% [7].

3. Toxic effects and fluorosis

High intake of fluoride may increase the risk of acute and chronic fluoride toxicity, fluorosis, and other systemic diseases. Some studies focus on the molecular mechanisms associated with fluoride toxicity. These studies have demonstrated that fluoride can induce oxidative stress, regulate intracellular redox homeostasis, lead to mitochondrial damage and endoplasmic reticulum stress, and alter gene expression [1, 2].

3.1 Acute toxicity

Taking a large amount of fluoride by mistake at one time can cause acute fluoride toxicity. The main symptoms are nausea, vomiting, diarrhea, and even intestinal bleeding. The serious ones cause organic damage, such as the heart, liver, and kidney, resulting in a coma. Patients usually die or recover within 4 h. It is a critical period; however it is very short. The principles of emergency treatment are emetic, gastric lavage, taking calcium orally or intravenously, sugar supplement, liquid supplement, and symptomatic treatment.

3.2 Chronic toxicity

Chronic fluoride toxicity can be caused by long-term excessive intake of fluoride. According to the different sources of fluoride, chronic fluoride toxicity can be divided into endemic fluorosis and industrial fluorosis. Firstly, endemic fluorosis is a kind of disease that occurs in a specific geographical environment. It is a chronic systemic accumulation of fluorosis caused by excessive intake of fluoride through water, air, or food. Drinking water with high concentration of fluoride and living with domestic coal pollution both may cause endemic fluorosis [8]. The degree of damage to the body mainly depends on the dose of fluoride. There is no significant difference in the effect of fluoride from different sources on the body. Secondly, industrial fluorosis usually exists in workers who work with cryolite and bauxite for a long time. They may intake excessive fluoride by eating, drinking, or breathing. The main clinical manifestations of chronic toxicity are dental fluorosis and skeletal fluorosis. Because dental fluorosis is manifested early in the cases of fluoride toxicity, dental fluorosis can be used as a biomarker of fluoride toxicity. Chronic exposure to excessive fluoride is associated with children's dental health and intelligence scores. A study found that dental fluorosis is positively related to the loss of high intelligence [9]. When it comes to how to prevent chronic fluorosis, there are three methods. First, the control of the concentration of fluoride in water. Water fluoridation is an effective way to prevent caries. However, the fluoride concentration should be monitored in case of dental fluorosis. As for those areas where the water has high content, it is necessary to take methods to remove fluoride from the water. Secondly, eliminate domestic coal pollution as much as possible. Last, the prevention of industrial fluoride pollution.

3.3 Dental fluorosis

Dental fluorosis is an excessive intake of fluoride during the mineralization period of tooth development. It is the most common sign of local chronic fluorosis, and it can be found early and quickly. Its clinical manifestations are as follows: (1) there are white strips on the surface of enamel, and the strips can fuse to form patches, even spread to the whole surface. (2) Some of the strips or plaques are yellowish or brown. (3) In severe cases, there is an enamel defect or tooth defect because of dental fluorosis.

Dental fluorosis mostly occurs in permanent teeth while less in primary teeth, because it is difficult for the fluoride to pass through the fetal blood barrier. The amount of teeth involved in dental fluorosis is related to the length of time living in the high-fluoride area during the tooth mineralization period. If a child moves in the high-fluoride zone after the age of 6–7, dental fluorosis almost does not appear. The severity of dental fluorosis depends on the degree of excessive intake of fluoride. If fluoride is severely excessive, the structure of enamel is disordered, and the tooth tends to stain or collapse. The principal reason of abnormal mineralization in dental fluorosis may be related to that high concentration of fluoride that can inhibit the activity of alkaline phosphatase, which is essential to bone and tooth formation.

The primary source of excessive fluoride intake is water fluoride [10]. Therefore, the principle of preventing dental fluorosis is avoiding absorbing excessive fluoride from water during the tooth mineralization period.

Some non-fluoride factors also may contribute to dental fluorosis. A research [11] discusses the effect of elemental contents on the risk of dental fluorosis, and it reported that high levels of F, Al, As, Pb, and Cr and low levels of Se, Zn, Cu, B, Ca, and P increase the risk of dental fluorosis. It suggests that taking measures to decrease the contents of F, Al, As, Pb, and Cr in the environment and increase the contents of Se, Zn, Cu, B, Ca, and P at the same time are useful for the control of fluorosis.

In addition, gene is regarded as a relevant risk factor of dental fluorosis [12]. Increasing evidence shows that an individual's genetic background could increase the risk of fluorosis when other factors like fluoride exposure remain the same [13]. A cross-sectional study [14] in Mexican children revealed an association of rs 412777 polymorphism in the COL1A2 gene with dental fluorosis. MMP20 was supposed to be related to the various phenotypes of dental fluorosis and may serve as a protective marker [15]. These would provide some evidence for identifying those people who are at risk of developing dental fluorosis in their later lives.

At the same time, we should pay attention to distinguishing dental fluorosis from enamel hypoplasia. Enamel hypoplasia usually has clear boundary strips and exists in one or more teeth. On the contrary, the strips of dental fluorosis have no definite boundary. The symptom regularly appears in several teeth, and patients often have a history of living in the high-fluoride area.

When it comes to how to treat dental fluorosis, bleaching and resin infiltration treatment both work for mild dental fluorosis [16]. However, for severe dental fluorosis, a full crown prosthesis is a better choice. A porcelain veneer is also used in severe cases [17]. Recently, some clinic studies discuss the effect of at-home bleaching and consider it effective and efficient [18]. Microabrasion is another hot topic. When removing the abnormal enamel affected by fluoride, it is necessary to protect the healthy tooth tissue as much as possible. Microabrasion not only can protect the healthy tooth tissue but also can achieve the aim of treating dental fluorosis [19].

3.4 Skeletal fluorosis

However, skeletal fluorosis may lead to the impairment of muscle movement, calcification of ligaments, increased osteosclerosis, and cancellous bone formation in the advanced stage. What's more, it may lead to the limitation of joint movement, muscle atrophy, and deformity of bone, spine, and major joints [2, 20].

4. Systemic use of fluoride

The correct way to use fluoride is that the body ingests fluoride through the digestive tract and passes through the gastrointestinal tract. The fluoride is absorbed into the blood circulation and then transferred to the tissues such as teeth and saliva to prevent caries. There are four main methods in the systemic use of fluoride, which are water fluoridation, salt fluoridation, milk fluoridation, and fluoride tablet.

4.1 Water fluoridation

Water fluoridation refers to adjusting the concentration of fluoride in water to appropriate level to prevent caries without causing the prevalence of dental fluorosis. Nowadays, water fluoridation is accepted by more than 150 science and health organization, such as the World Health Organization (WHO) and the International Association for Dental Research (IADR) [4, 10, 21]. In 1958, Singapore was the first country in Asia to carry out water fluoridation, which covers 100% of its population. It does contribute to improving the level of oral health in Singapore [22]. Some researchers assessed disability-adjusted life years (DALYs) and DALY rate due to dental caries preventable through water fluoridation in Iran, and they found that in 2016 DALYs were 14,971 (95% uncertainty interval 7348–24,725) and DALY rate was 18.73 (9.19–30.93) [23]. The results indicated that water fluoridation plays an important role in dental public health at the national level. According to the WHO's recommendation, the allowed fluoride level in water is 1.5 mg/L.

4.2 Salt fluoridation

Unlike water fluoridation, the carrier of salt fluoridation is salt. Fluoride is added into salt and is absorbed into the body by eating salt. It is reported the salt fluoridation was used in a dental research project in Colombia [24], and now it is extended into more than 20 countries [4]. Although salt fluoridation is not as popular as water fluoridation, it is still a supplement to water fluoridation, especially in the low-fluoride area and no tap water area. The dietary habit is different in different countries; therefore, the amount of salt intake in different countries is different. Thus, the content of added fluoride ought to depend on specific conditions.

Although salt fluoridation is not restricted by water service, the most disadvantaged point of this method is that the fluoride content is precisely hard to control. If someone prefers to eat salty, it is more likely for him/her to get dental fluorosis, which causes caries. What's more, considering that few citizens know about how much fluoride was added into salt, the government participating in water fluoride is a better choice.

4.3 Milk fluoridation

Milk fluoridation is another way to use fluoride, which means the fluoride is added into milk or milk powder. However, it has the same shortcoming as salt fluoridation—difficult to control. Milk is considered containing nutrients that help to buffer acid, and it may reduce the risk of dental caries after exposure to a sugar beverage. A research studied the effect of rinsing with water, non-fluoridated milk, and fluoridated milk on acidic dental plaque, the results showed that rinsing with fluoridated milk increased the pH value of acidic plaque to the resting level faster [25]. Considering the safety of using fluoride, the intake of fluoride should be controlled strictly. Therefore, the propaganda and education of milk fluoridation are important.

4.4 Fluoride tablet

Fluoride tablet is a supplementary method of systemic application of fluoride for children, especially for the children who live in the area with low content of fluoride, and when the government does not carry out water fluoridation policy. Fluoride tablet must be used under dentists' recommendations and teachers' or parents' supervision. A study assessed adherence to oral fluoride and barriers to adherence in a community without water fluoridation, and more than half of parents were found that they either had not or did not know whether their children had received fluoride on the day before. What's more, adherence to fluoride tablets in the primary care setting is low [26]. If possible, choosing water fluoridation as a systemic fluoride application method is a better choice.

5. Topical application of fluoride

The topical way to use fluoride is to apply fluoride directly to the surface of the tooth. It is a double-edged sword. On the one hand, this method can increase the topical concentration of fluoride quickly and make fluoride play a better role in prevention and treatment. At the same time, topical use is a supplement to the systemic use of fluoride. The combination of these two methods will enhance the effect of fluoride. On the other hand, higher topical fluoride concentration may cause toxic effects, such as dental fluorosis. And fluoride can enter the digestive tract through the oral cavity, and then it will be absorbed into the blood, resulting in toxic effects.

However, if we use fluoride in the right way, we can avoid the toxic effects of fluoride almost completely. So, it is important to know how to use fluoride in a correct way.

The common ways to use fluoride topically are through fluoride toothpaste, fluoride mouth rinse, fluoride varnish, fluoride gel, and fluoride foam. They will be explained separately.

5.1 Fluoride toothpaste

There are many different types of toothpastes on the market that are applied to prevent caries and improve oral health. Around 90% of these contain fluoride, a mineral found in relatively low concentrations in fresh and seawater. Fluoride toothpaste by far provides a higher level of the mineral than any other source. It is a cheap and convenient way to promote dental health, which is recognized by the Centers for Disease Control and Prevention to be "one of 10 great public health achievements of the 20th century."

There are different kinds of fluoride toothpaste, such as sodium fluoride toothpaste and stannous fluoride toothpaste. It is generally believed that fluoride toothpaste has a noticeable effect on caries prevention [27, 28].

5.1.1 Sodium fluoride toothpaste

It is crucial to keep the activity of fluoride ion in sodium fluoride toothpaste. In the earlier year, due to the incompatibility of sodium fluoride with calcium carbonate, calcium phosphate, and other friction agents in toothpaste, the fluoride ion lost its activity, and the prevention effect was not evident [29]. However, after the reasonable selection of friction agents, such as acrylic plastic, calcium pyrophosphate, or silica, it is proven that the control effect is positive. Nowadays, sodium fluoride toothpaste is popular, and it does not have the defect of staining teeth.

5.1.2 Stannous fluoride

Stannous fluoride toothpaste can not only prevent caries but also provide antibacterial function and provide relief from dentin hypersensitivity [30]. The researchers studied the action mode of stannous and sodium fluoride toothpaste on anti-biofilm properties. The results revealed that stannous fluoride toothpaste had a better antibacterial effect on microbial biofilm. And stannous fluoride toothpaste was able to regulate microbial composition within a multi-species biofilm [31]. However, long-term use of stannous fluoride toothpaste could lead to tooth staining [32]. The tooth discoloration caused by stannous fluoride is due to the reaction of the tooth with the tin ion present in the formulation. And stannous ion may also cause the toothpaste to taste bad. At the same time, the stannous ion easily loses its activity in toothpaste.

Recently, researchers try to find a new formula. First of all, the composite chelating technology can stabilize the stannous ion in the toothpaste effectively during the storage and transportation processes. Moreover, the stannous ion still can be released rapidly during the brushing process. Meanwhile, the stannous ion is stabilized by the composite chelating technology to resist the staining problem of stannous fluoride. It was reported that the addition of zinc phosphate could significantly improve the stability of stannous ion more effectively than other stabilization methods [33].

Besides, researchers are looking for more effective fluoride toothpaste to prevent caries. A study showed that the incorporation of 2% arginine in sodium fluoride toothpaste significantly increased the remineralization of enamel caries-like lesion when compared to sodium fluoride toothpaste [34].

5.2 Fluoride mouth rinse

When fluoride is added into mouth rinse, we call it fluoride mouth rinse. Although mouth rinse only stays in the oral cavity for a short time, it is still considered as having an effect on the prevention of caries. As reported, the combined use of fluoride toothpaste and mouth rinse shows better results than the use of either alone [35]. The most commonly used fluoride mouth rinse is sodium fluoride mouth rinse. Fluoride mouth rinse is suitable for those people who have a high risk of dental caries, who are in orthodontic treatment with a fixed appliance, or who can't take care of themselves. Because of its advantages, like low price, easy to master, and convenient to use, it is an excellent choice for school-age children. It is also necessary to read the instruction on how to use mouth rinse carefully, especially when children use it. The dose of fluoride should be controlled strictly, and mouth rinse could not be drunk. So the compliance of children needs to be taken into account.

5.3 Fluoride varnish

Fluoride varnish has a higher fluoride concentration than fluoride toothpaste and fluoride mouth rinse. It can be more durable on the surface of the tooth. There are more than 30 fluoride varnish products on the market today, most of which could be classified into 2.26% fluoride and 0.1% fluoride varnish categories [28]. It should be used with dentists' professional judgment and applied in a dental clinic or hospital. After the curing of fluoride varnish, the tooth will discolor temporarily, but brushing the tooth will make tooth return to previous color.

5.4 Fluoride gel and fluoride foam

Fluoride gel and fluoride foam both have a higher content of fluoride. Acidulated phosphate fluoride (APF) gel or foam is a universal fluoride gel or foam. As for fluoride gel, it contains many kinds of gels with different fluoride concentrations. Some of them are allowed to be used by individuals, but others should be used by professionals. The operation method shall be in accordance with the direction. Fluoride foam can inhibit the formation of caries. Therefore, the dose of fluoride foam is much less than the same effective concentration fluoride gel.

5.5 Recommendations for professional topical fluoride application

Whether using topical fluoride or not should be judged by professionals. And individual patient's preferences should also be taken into account.

According to the recommendations provided by the American Dental Association (ADA) [28], people who are at risk of developing dental caries could take the following topical fluorides: fluoride varnish, fluoride gel, fluoride mouth rinse, and fluoride toothpaste. 2.26% fluoride varnish was recommended for people older than 6 years for both coronal and root caries. Some studies showed that there was no benefit of 0.1% fluoride varnish application in children younger than 6 years. The ADA only recommended 2.26% fluoride varnish for children younger than 6 years because of the low risk of caries, although other topical fluorides may have some evidence of a benefit. As for fluoride gel, 1.23% fluoride (acidulated phosphate fluoride) gel was confirmed beneficial to younger than 6 and 6–18 age groups. It could also produce an effect on adult root caries prevention. However, the potential harm associated with swallowing APF gel could outweigh these benefits. That is why 1.23% fluoride gel was not recommended for children younger than 6 years. When it comes to fluoride foam, it shouldn't be applied to children under 6 years, and the reason is the same as the fluoride gel. There was a kind of prescription-strength, home-use gel mentioned in ADA's recommendations, which was 0.5% fluoride gel. Researchers judged that the benefits of fluoride gel in older than 6 age groups outweighed potential harm. Prescription-strength, home-use mouth rinse contains 0.09% fluoride, and its benefit outweighs the potential harm. In conclusion, 2.26% fluoride varnish or 1.23% fluoride gel or a prescription-strength, home-use 0.5% fluoride gel or 0.09% fluoride mouth rinse is all recommended for patients 6 years or older. Only 2.26% fluoride varnish is recommended for children younger than 6 years.

5.6 Recommendations of topical fluoride application for different ages

People of different caries risk levels need different caries prevention methods [27]. Children under the age of 6 years who have any incipient or cavitated primary or secondary carious lesion during the last 3 years or have a suboptimal fluoride exposure or xerostomia should be classified as having a high risk of caries. Socioeconomic status can also be an essential factor. In terms of anyone older than 6 years, the standard of caries amount is expanded to three or more incipient or cavitated primary or secondary carious lesions in the last 3 years. No incipient or cavitated primary or secondary carious lesions during the previous 3 years and no factors that may increase caries risk (see Appendix for details) are a standard of low caries risk for any ages.

Generally, fluoride toothpaste is recommended for almost everyone. However, it should be noticed that children need a lower dose of fluoride toothpaste [36].

5.6.1 Younger than 6 years

Low-risk patients in this group may receive no benefit from topical fluoride application. Fluoride toothpaste may provide them adequate prevention. High-risk patients should receive fluoride varnish applications at 3- to 6-month intervals.

5.6.2 Six to 18 years of age

Low-risk patients do not need professional topical fluoride application. Higher-risk patients should receive fluoride varnish or gel application at 6-month intervals. Fluoride varnish applications every 3 months or fluoride gels every 3 months may provide additional caries prevention benefit.

5.6.3 Older than 18 years

For lower-risk patients, whether to apply topical fluoride or not is a decision that should balance the consideration with the professional judgment and the individual patient's preferences. Higher-risk patients should receive fluoride varnish or gel applications each 3–6 months.

As for fluoride foam, it is commonly used in practice. The evidence of its effectiveness is not as strong as the fluoride gel and varnish. But it does provide the benefit of lower fluoride dose than fluoride gel.

Conflict of interest

The authors declare no conflict of interest.

Appendix

According to the recommendations of the American Dental Association (ADA), the topical application of fluoride should take caries risk status into consideration. The caries risk criteria are as follows:

Patients should be evaluated using caries risk criteria such as those below.
Low caries risk
All age groups
No incipient or cavitated primary or secondary carious lesions during the last 3 years and no factors that may increase caries risk*
Moderate caries risk
Younger than 6 years
No incipient or cavitated primary or secondary carious lesions during the last 3 years but presence of at least one factor that may increase caries risk*
Older than 6 years (any of the following)
One or two incipient or cavitated primary or secondary carious lesions in the last 3 years.
No incipient or cavitated primary or secondary carious lesions in the last 3 years but presence of at least one factor that may increase caries risk*
High caries risk
Younger than 6 years (any of the following)
Any incipient or cavitated primary or secondary carious lesion during the last 3 years
Presence of multiple factors that may increase caries risk*
Low socioeconomic status†
Suboptimal fluoride exposure
Xerostomia‡
Older than 6 years (any of the following)
Three or more incipient or cavitated primary or secondary carious lesions in the last 3 years
Presence of multiple factors that may increase caries risk*
Suboptimal fluoride exposure
Xerostomia‡

**Factors increasing risk of developing caries also may include, but are not limited to, high titers of cariogenic bacteria, poor oral hygiene, prolonged nursing (bottle or breast), poor family dental health, developmental or acquired enamel defects, genetic abnormality of teeth, many multisurface restorations, chemotherapy or radiation therapy, eating disorders, drug or alcohol abuse, irregular dental care, cariogenic diet, active orthodontic treatment, presence of exposed root surfaces, restoration overhangs and open margins, and physical or mental disability with inability or unavailability of performing proper oral health care.*
†On the basis of findings from population studies, groups with low socioeconomic status have been found to have an increased risk of developing caries. In children too young for their risk to be based on caries history, low socioeconomic status should be considered as a caries risk factor.
‡Medication-, radiation-, or disease-induced xerostomia.

Author details

Haiyang Sun[1,2], Feng Luo[1,2]* and Qianbing Wan[1,2]

1 Department of Prosthodontics, West China Hospital of Stomatology, Sichuan University, Chengdu, China

2 State Key Laboratory of Oral Diseases, National Clinical Research Center for Oral Diseases, West China Hospital of Stomatology, Sichuan University, Chengdu, China

*Address all correspondence to: luofeng0122@icloud.com

References

[1] Zohoori FV, Duckworth RM. Chapter 44—Fluoride: Intake and metabolism, therapeutic and toxicological consequences. In: Collins JF, editor. Molecular, Genetic, and Nutritional Aspects of Major and Trace Minerals. Boston: Academic Press; 2017. pp. 539-550. DOI: 10.1016/B978-0-12-802168-2.00044-0

[2] Thompson LJ. Chapter 27—Fluoride. In: Gupta RC, editor. Veterinary Toxicology. 3rd ed.: Academic Press; 2018. pp. 429-431. DOI: 10.1016/B978-0-12-811410-0.00027-1

[3] Wang M, Li X, He W, Li J, Zhu Y, Liao Y, et al. Distribution, health risk assessment, and anthropogenic sources of fluoride in farmland soils in phosphate industrial area, southwest China. Environmental Pollution. 2019;**249**:423-433. DOI: 10.1016/j.envpol.2019.03.044

[4] Hu D et al. The Preventive Dentistry. 6th ed.: People's Medical Publishing House; 2012

[5] Huang W, Shahid S, Anderson P. 25—Applications of silver diamine fluoride in management of dental caries. In: Khurshid Z, Najeeb S, Zafar MS, Sefat F, editors. Advanced Dental Biomaterials. Woodhead Publishing; 2019. pp. 675-699. DOI: 10.1016/B978-0-08-102476-8.00023-2

[6] Yu OY, Zhao IS, Mei ML, Lo ECM, Chu CH. Caries—Arresting effects of silver diamine fluoride and sodium fluoride on dentine caries lesions. Journal of Dentistry. 2018;**78**:65-71. DOI: 10.1016/j.jdent.2018.08.007

[7] Gold J. Silver diamine fluoride may prevent and arrest root caries in older adults. The Journal of Evidence-Based Dental Practice. 2019;**19**(2):186-188. DOI: 10.1016/j.jebdp.2019.05.009

[8] Yuan L, Fei W, Jia F, Jun-ping L, Qi L, Fang-ru N, et al. Health risk in children to fluoride exposure in a typical endemic fluorosis area on Loess Plateau, north China, in the last decade. Chemosphere. 2020;**243**:125451. DOI: 10.1016/j.chemosphere.2019.125451

[9] Yu X, Chen J, Li Y, Liu H, Hou C, Zeng Q, et al. Threshold effects of moderately excessive fluoride exposure on children's health: A potential association between dental fluorosis and loss of excellent intelligence. Environment International. 2018;**118**:116-124. DOI: 10.1016/j.envint.2018.05.042

[10] Mandinic Z, Curcic M, Antonijevic B, Carevic M, Mandic J, Djukic-Cosic D, et al. Fluoride in drinking water and dental fluorosis. Science of the Total Environment. 2010;**408**(17):3507-3512. DOI: 10.1016/j.scitotenv.2010.04.029

[11] Xu Y, Huang H, Zeng Q, Yu C, Yao M, Hong F, et al. The effect of elemental content on the risk of dental fluorosis and the exposure of the environment and population to fluoride produced by coal-burning. Envrionmental Toxicology and Pharmacology. 2017;**56**:329-339. DOI: 10.1016/j.etap.2017.10.011

[12] Pramanik S, Saha D. The genetic influence in fluorosis. Envrionmental Toxicology and Pharmacology. 2017;**56**:157-162. DOI: 10.1016/j.etap.2017.09.008

[13] Rahila C, Aswath Narayanan MB, Ramesh Kumar SG, Leena Selvamary A, Sujatha A, John KJ. Association of COL1A2 (PvuII) gene polymorphism with risk and severity of dental fluorosis—A case control study. The Saudi Dental Journal. 2019;**31**(4):463-468. DOI: 10.1016/j.sdentj.2019.05.004

[14] Jarquín-Yñezá L, Alegría-Torres JA, Castillo CG, de Jesús Mejía-Saavedra J. Dental fluorosis and a polymorphism in the COL1A2 gene in Mexican children. Archives of Oral Biology. 2018;**96**:21-25. DOI: 10.1016/j.archoralbio.2018.08.010

[15] Tremillo-Maldonado O, Molina-Frechero N, González-González R, Damián-Matsumura P, Sánchez-Pérez L, Sicco E, et al. DNA sequencing reveals AMELX, ODAM and MMP20 variations in dental fluorosis. Archives of Oral Biology. 2020;**110**:104626. DOI: 10.1016/j.archoralbio.2019.104626

[16] Castro KS, de Araújo Ferreira AC, Duarte RM, Sampaio FC, Meireles SS. Acceptability, efficacy and safety of two treatment protocols for dental fluorosis: A randomized clinical trial. Journal of Dentistry. 2014;**42**(8):938-944. DOI: 10.1016/j.jdent.2014.01.011

[17] Slaska B, Liebman AI, Kukleris D. Restoration of fluorosis stained teeth: A case study. Dental Clinics of North America. 2015;**59**(3):583-591. DOI: 10.1016/j.cden.2015.03.003

[18] Pan Z, Que K, Liu J, Sun G, Chen Y, Wang L, et al. Effects of at-home bleaching and resin infiltration treatments on the aesthetic and psychological status of patients with dental fluorosis: A prospective study. Journal of Dentistry. 2019;**91**:103228. DOI: 10.1016/j.jdent.2019.103228

[19] Romero MF, Babb CS, Delash J, Brackett WW. Minimally invasive esthetic improvement in a patient with dental fluorosis by using microabrasion and bleaching: A clinical report. The Journal of Prosthetic Dentistry. 2018;**120**(3):323-326. DOI: 10.1016/j.prosdent.2017.12.024

[20] Daiwile AP, Tarale P, Sivanesan S, Naoghare PK, Bafana A, Parmar D, et al. Role of fluoride induced epigenetic alterations in the development of skeletal fluorosis. Ecotoxicology and Environmental Safety. 2019;**169**:410-417. DOI: 10.1016/j.ecoenv.2018.11.035

[21] Egor M, Birungi G. Fluoride contamination and its optimum upper limit in groundwater from Sukulu Hills, Tororo District, Uganda. Scientific African. 2020;**7**:e241. DOI: 10.1016/j.sciaf.2019.e00241

[22] Chong GTF, Tseng P. A review of the uses of fluoride and outcomes of dental caries control in Singapore. Singapore Dental Journal. 2011;**32**(1):14-148. DOI: 10.1016/S0377-5291(12)70011-1

[23] Abtahi M, Dobaradaran S, Jorfi S, Koolivand A, Mohebbi MR, Montazeri A, et al. Age-sex specific and sequela-specific disability-adjusted life years (DALYs) due to dental caries preventable through water fluoridation: An assessment at the national and subnational levels in Iran, 2016. Environmental Research. 2018;**167**:372-385. DOI: 10.1016/j.envres.2018.08.005

[24] Fluoridated salt used in dental research project in Colombia. The Journal of the American Dental Association. 1967;**75**(3):582-584. DOI: 10.14219/jada.archive.1967.0270

[25] Jirarattanasopha V, Pruetpongpun N, Amornpipithkul C, Sanguansin S. Effect of nonfluoridated milk and fluoridated milk on acidic dental plaque. Pediatric Dental Journal. 2019;**29**(2):53-58. DOI: 10.1016/j.pdj.2019.06.001

[26] Flood SM, Asplund KB, Hoffman BM, Nye AB, Zuckerman KMM. Fluoride supplementation adherence and barriers in a community without water fluoridation. Academic Pediatrics. 2016;**17**(3):316-322. DOI: 10.1016/j.acap.2016.11.009

[27] American Dental Association Council on Scientific Affairs. Professionally applied topical: Evidence-based clinical recommendations. The Journal of the American Dental

Association. 2006;**137**(8):1151-1159. DOI: 10.14219/jada.archive.2006.0356

[28] Weyant RJ, Tracy SL, Anselmo TT, Beltrán-Aguilar ED, Donly KJ, Frese WA, et al. Topical fluoride for caries prevention. The Journal of the American Dental Association. 2013;**144**(11):1279-1291. DOI: 10.14219/jada.archive.2013.0057

[29] Hattab FN. The state of fluorides in toothpastes. Journal of Dentistry. 1989;**17**(2):47-54. DOI: 10.1016/0300-5712(89)90129-2

[30] Hines D, Xu S, Stranick M, Lavender S, Pilch S, Zhang Y, et al. Effect of a stannous fluoride toothpaste on dentinal hypersensitivity: In vitro and clinical evaluation. The Journal of the American Dental Association. 2019;**150**(4 Suppl):S47-S59. DOI: 10.1016/j.adaj.2019.01.006

[31] Cheng X, Liu J, Li J, Zhou X, Wang L, Liu J, et al. Comparative effect of a stannous fluoride toothpaste and a sodium fluoride toothpaste on a multispecies biofilm. Archives of Oral Biology. 2017;**74**:5-11. DOI: 10.1016/j.archoralbio.2016.10.030

[32] Mason S, Young S, Qaqish J, Frappin G, Goyal C. Stain control with two modified stannous fluoride/sodium tripolyphosphate toothpastes: A randomised controlled proof of concept study. Journal of Dentistry. 2019;**2**:100009. DOI: 10.1016/j.jjodo.2019.100009

[33] Myers CP, Pappas I, Makwana E, Begum-Gafur R, Utgikar N, Alsina MA, et al. Solving the problem with stannous fluoride: Formulation, stabilization, and antimicrobial action. The Journal of the American Dental Association. 2019;**150**(4 Suppl):S5-S13. DOI: 10.1016/j.adaj.2019.01.004

[34] Bijle MNA, Ekambaram M, Lo EC, Yiu CKY. The combined enamel remineralization potential of arginine and fluoride toothpaste. Journal of Dentistry. 2018;**76**:75-82. DOI: 10.1016/j.jdent.2018.06.009

[35] Carvalho TS, Lussi A. Combined effect of a fluoride-, stannous- and chitosan-containing toothpaste and stannous-containing rinse on the prevention of initial enamel erosion–abrasion. Journal of Dentistry. 2014;**42**(4):450-459. DOI: 10.1016/j.jdent.2014.01.004

[36] Wright JT, Hanson N, Ristic H, Whall CW, Estrich CG, et al. Fluoride toothpaste efficacy and safety in children younger than 6 years: A systematic review. Journal of the American Dental Association. 2014;**145**(2):182-189. DOI: 10.14219/jada.2013.37

Chapter 6

The Use of Silver Diamine Fluoride in Pediatric Dentistry

Ana Cláudia Rodrigues Chibinski

Abstract

This book chapter aims to discuss the main aspects related to the use of silver diamine fluoride (SDF) in Pediatric Dentistry. The composition and mechanism of action of the SDF are presented, as well as the application technique and indications. The effectiveness of SDF is reported based on contemporary scientific evidence from laboratory and clinical studies, focusing on its effect in enamel and dentin remineralization and caries arrestment. Parental and professional acceptance of tooth staining is presented, as well as the use of potassium iodide as a possible alternative to manage this side-effect. Taking all the discussed information together, it is possible to conclude that the SDF is a simple and effective treatment to halt the dental caries progress in children.

Keywords: silver diamine fluoride, dental caries, child, Pediatric Dentistry, tooth remineralization

1. Introduction

Untreated caries lesions in deciduous teeth affect more than 570 million children around the world. One very disturbing evidence is that the prevalence of untreated caries lesion remained stable from 1990 to 2015 [1] and the peak of the disease is among very young children, aging 1–4 years old [2].

Dental caries is a dynamic, multifactorial, non-communicable and biofilm-mediated disease. It has a very strong behavioral component, with a direct influence of diet and hygiene habits. When there is an imbalance in the biological, behavioral, and environmental factors, carious lesions will develop [3].

Therefore, alternative treatment strategies are needed to modify this scenario. First of all, one should be aware that dental caries is a preventable disease, that can be controlled by reducing the amount of fermentable carbohydrates available in the diet and by disorganizing the dental biofilm systematically [4]. However, if these simple and effective measures fail, carious lesions may develop and they should be treated according to the Minimal Invasive Dentistry philosophy. The management of these lesions depends on the invasiveness of the lesion (in enamel or dentin) and the degree of tissue removal associated with the procedure. It includes dietary and biofilm control, mineralization techniques, sealing, restorative techniques and non-restorative techniques [5].

Currently, a non-invasive agent has received renewed interest: silver diamine fluoride (SDF). It is an efficient, affordable, equitable and effective cariostatic agent. This non-restorative approach can halt the progression of carious lesions and it can be an alternative to control the burden of dental caries in children around the world [6]. This is an interesting treatment approach for deciduous teeth that is recommended by the American Academy of Pediatric Dentistry, that published a guideline, in 2017, named "Use of Silver Diamine Fluoride for Dental Caries Management in Children and Adolescents, Including Those with Special Health Care Needs" [7].

The use of SDF for arresting dental caries in deciduous and permanent teeth is not a novelty in Dentistry. Since the 1970s, when it was developed, it has been widely used in Japan, as well as in other countries such as Brazil, Argentina, China, and Australia [8]. Notwithstanding, it was not commonly used in the United States of America until 2014, when the use of SDF was cleared by the Food and Drug Administration (FDA) as an agent to treat tooth hypersensitivity and, in an off-label indication, for caries arrestment management.

A significant number of randomized clinical trials ascertain the usefulness of SDF for Pediatric Dentistry, aiming to control and/or arresting dental caries in deciduous teeth [9–13] and first permanent molars [14, 15].

This chapter will guide clinicians regarding the use of diamine silver fluoride in their daily practice, using a critical appraisal of the available scientific literature regarding its action mechanism, effectiveness, and child/parent acceptance. This theoretical approach is in concordance with evidence-based dentistry and will enable the professional to understand the benefits and shortcomings behind the use of SDF in Pediatric Dentistry.

2. Composition and action mechanisms: how does SDF work in a carious lesion?

SDF ($AgF[NH_3]_2$) is a colorless solution with alkaline pH (pH 8–10). Its main components are silver, fluoride and ammonia. Basically, the silver is an antimicrobial agent, the ammonia stabilizes the solution, while the fluoride aids remineralization [16]. Nevertheless, the action mechanisms of SDF is much more complex as it will be shown hereinafter.

The most common concentration is 38%, which represents 44.800 ppm of fluoride and 255.000 ppm of silver [17]. These two elements, in such a high concentration, will have a synergistic activity, with a bactericidal action on cariogenic microorganisms, promotion of mineralization, inhibition of demineralization of tooth hard tissues, and decrease of the destruction of the organic portion of the dentin [18]. Other concentrations of SDF (10, 12, 30%) are available in Brazil from different manufacturers. **Table 1** shows the commercially available brands of SDF.

When SDF is applied to the tooth, the following reaction occurs:

$$Ca_{10}(PO_4)_6(OH)_2 + Ag(NH_3)_2F \rightarrow CaF_2 + Ag_3PO_4 + NH_4OH$$

$$(\text{hydroxyapatite} + \text{SDF} \rightarrow \text{calcium fluoride} + \text{silver phosphate} + \text{ammonium hydroxide})$$

The main action of fluoride is related to the remineralization of the dental hard tissues. After SDF application on a carious lesion, two compounds are formed: calcium fluoride and fluorhydroxyapatite. Calcium fluoride is loosely bound to the teeth and it can be considered a reservoir of fluoride that will be released if a pH

Trademark (manufacturer)	Country	SDF concentration	Commercial appearance
Advantage arrest (Elevate Oral Care)	EUA	38%	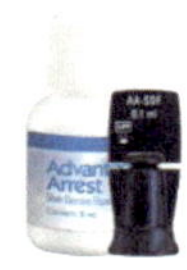
Cariostasul (Iodontosul)	Brazil	10, 12 and 30%	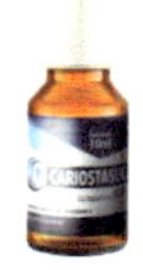
Cariestop (Biodinâmica Química eFarmacêutica SRL)	Brazil	12 and 30%	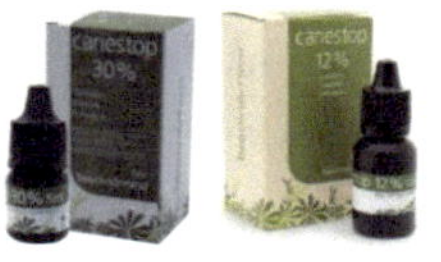
Ancarie (Maquira)	Brazil	12%	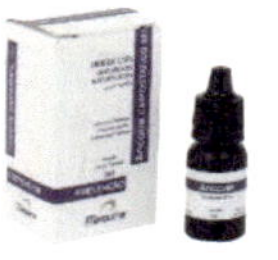
Fagamin (Tedequim SRL)	Argentina	38%	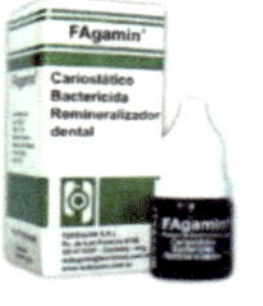
Fluoroplat (NAF Laboratórios)	Argentina	38%	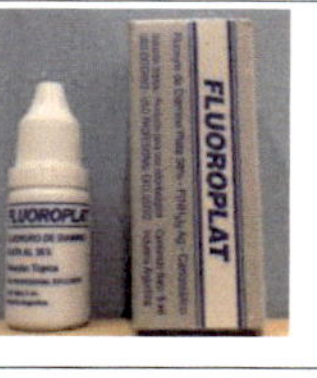
Saforide (Toyo Seiyaku Kasei Co. Ltda)	Japan	38%	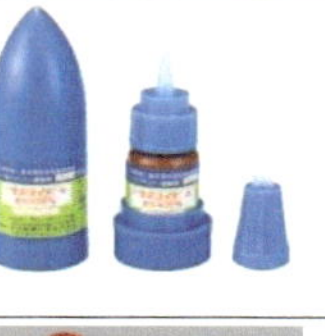
CSDS - Caries Status Disclosing Solution (Creighton Dental)	Australia	40%	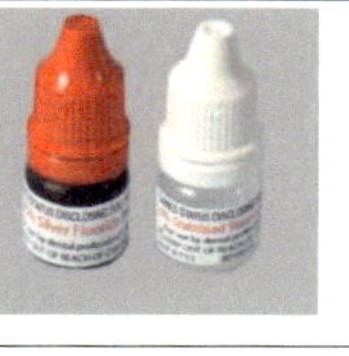
e-SDF (Kids-e-dental)	India	38%	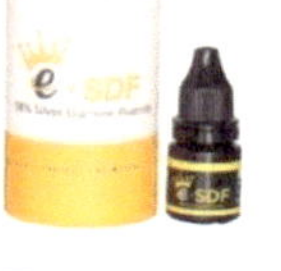

Trademark (manufacturer)	Country	SDF concentration	Commercial appearance
Riva Star (SDI Dental Limited)	Australia	38%	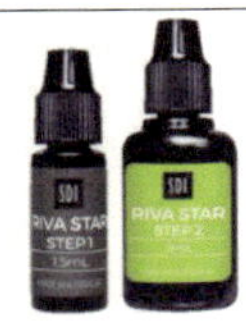

Table 1.
SDF products available in different countries.

drop occurs; therefore, there will be available fluoride during the DES-RE process. Silver phosphate can also act as a reservoir of phosphate ions for the next caries challenge [19].

The fluorhydroxyapatite is formed when fluoride is incorporated into the hydroxyapatite crystals; it helps remineralization and makes the tooth more resistant to further demineralization [18, 20]. Also, high concentration of fluorides can inhibit the formation of biofilm, since fluoride can influence the carbohydrate metabolism and the sugar uptake of the microorganisms [8]. The silver ions (Ag^{+}) exert a great antimicrobial effect, killing or interfering in the microorganisms' metabolic processes [8]. There are different mechanisms involved in this effect. Silver ions can bind to the cell-wall structure and inhibit the mobility of the bacteria or promote the rupture of the membranes. They also can form organometallic complexes inside the bacterial cell, liberating silver ions that will interact with the DNA of the microorganisms, resulting in inactivation of bacterial DNA/RNA or mutation of the DNA, leading to the death of the bacteria [20].

However, the progression of a carious lesion evolves not only the demineralization of the enamel and dentin as a result of bacterial acids, but also the destruction of the organic content of the dentin, composed mainly by type I collagen (around 90%). The loss of dentin minerals exposes the organic matrix, which is degraded by bacterial and host-derived enzymes [21]. Maintenance of the collagen fibrils is important because it acts as a scaffold for the deposition of mineral crystals [22] and might inhibit the diffusion of calcium and phosphate for further demineralization. Therefore, it is very important for the arrestment of a carious lesion that SDF can also exert inhibitory effects on the degradation of dentin collagen fibrils by inactivating the endogenous metalloproteinases and cathepsins [23].

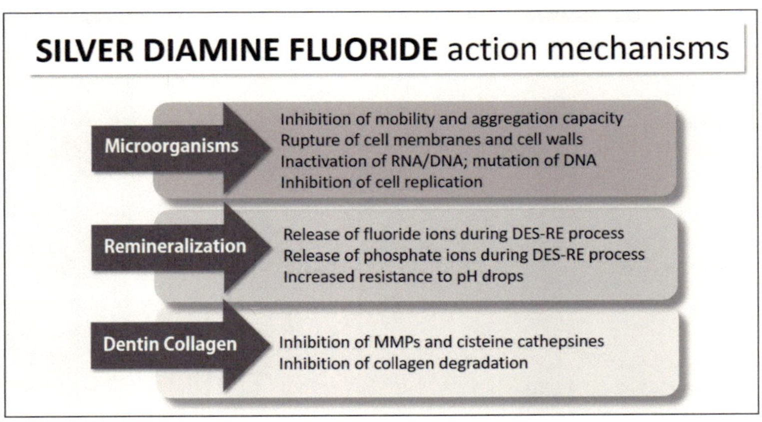

Figure 1.
Silver diamine fluoride action mechanisms [8, 20, 23, 24].

For descriptive purposes only, the action of each SDF compound was presented apart. Notwithstanding, the effectiveness of SDF is a result of the combination of fluoride and silver ions and they occur simultaneously (**Figure 1**).

3. Why use SDF? Indications, advantages, and disadvantages

SDF is an effective, safe, and equitable product [25]. It offers the clinician the possibility of avoiding invasive treatments and the use of dental local anesthesia and dental drills, which triggers for dental fear and anxiety. In young patients with behavioral problems that cannot be manageable in a normal clinical setting, the option for an SDF treatment may avoid sedation and general anesthesia and the risks associated with them.

The low cost and the simplicity of the treatment make the use of SDF an interesting option to provide oral care for vulnerable populations, without regular access to dental health professional or in Public Health Dentistry. It can also be considered an inclusive treatment, since it may be used in a large range of patients. Due to its facility of application, the treatment with SDF can be accomplished in a dental office, but also at alternative venues like daycares facilities for children, hospitals, and nursing homes.

As a non-invasive and non-restorative procedure, SDF is a smart choice if the dentist wants to arrest active carious processes quickly, in deciduous and permanent teeth, and create the time to improve the oral conditions without worsening the clinical signs of the disease. At this moment, the patient may be stimulated to modify wrongful dietary and oral hygiene practices and oral homeostasis may be obtained. Simultaneously, the carious lesions will be arrested, and, if the patient/parents want to improve form or esthetics, further restorative treatment may be accomplished in a more responsive and positive environment. Anyway, restoration is not paramount to maintain health.

In Pediatric Dentistry, the extra time obtained with the use of SDF may also be fundamental to improve the behavior of the patients and their ability to cope with the dentist during the dental treatment [24]. Besides that, the main indications are listed as follows and includes patients that have [26]:

- early childhood caries;
- behavioral problems (SDF is an alternative to sedation or general anesthesia treatment);
- special needs like severe cognitive or physical disabilities;
- dental phobia or those who cannot tolerate standard dental treatment for medical or psychological reasons, including pre-cooperative children;
- multiple cavitated active lesions that need immediate intervention to avoid the progression of the carious lesions, that can become symptomatic while waiting for the completion of the traditional restorative treatment;
- extensive lesions that are too extensive to restore and are not associated with spontaneous pain and/or infection.

Regarding the tooth, the application of SDF will only be possible in the absence of clinical signs of pulpal inflammation, spontaneous or nocturnal toothache, and pulp exposition [7].

SDF can also be used in enamel lesions, to control proximal carious lesions in deciduous teeth [27], and to arrest incipient occlusal caries in erupting permanent first molars [14].

The use of SDF is contraindicated in patients who have a history of silver allergy, since it may cause gingivitis or mucositis [26].

The staining of the tooth is the main disadvantage of SDF usage. It is expected that carious tissue in enamel and dentin will become dark brown or black after application. Parents and patients must be aware that the staining is the clinical sign of the arrestment of the carious lesion, that the stain will remain over time, and that its removal will only be possible with the use of burs. Sound enamel will not be stained.

4. What about the concentration and periodicity of application?

The current literature recommends the use of 38% SDF solution [10, 12, 22, 28], with two annual application (every 6 months) [13, 28, 29], without previous removal of carious tissue [26].

This recommendation is based on randomized clinical trials, that focused on the effectiveness of SDF in arresting or inactivating carious lesions in dentin in deciduous teeth. Data from different studies [10, 12] comprehended a total of 1864 patients, that were followed-up from 24 [12] to 30 months [10]. The concentrations of 12 and 38% SDF were compared, and the 38% SDF was consistently more effective than 12% in inactivating carious lesions in prescholars [10, 12, 28].

The annual application of SDF 38% is effective in arresting dentin carious lesions. However, increased frequency of application will raise the caries arrest rates by about 15%. It was shown that the caries arrest rates of 38% SDF were 66.9% for annual application and 75.7% for semiannual application [10].

4.1 Additional information

Other variables regarding individual characteristics of the patients should be considered when choosing SDF concentration and periodicity.

Children's oral hygiene is the most important one since there is a significant interaction between frequency/efficacy of SDF application and oral hygiene status [10]. Children at high caries risk, as reflected by their high mean baseline dmfs and plaque scores, may not achieve the expected results with the exclusive use of SDF, even at a concentration of 38%. Therefore, these patients will be highly benefited by the biannual application of this solution at 38%.

There is also an interaction between the SDF concentration and the lesion site. The combination of lesion site and SDF concentration should be taken into consideration when applying SDF solution for caries arrest, and 38% SDF should always be used, particularly in posterior teeth [28]. Cavities that show a retentive design may provide sites for dental biofilm retention and may difficult the contact with fluoride dentifrice and toothbrush on a daily basis; this is more probable to occur in cavities of posterior teeth.

At the surface level, SDF treatments on smooth surfaces of anterior teeth as well as on the buccal or lingual tooth surfaces had a higher chance to become arrested [13].

To overcome these minor setbacks, the SDF treatment, as any other dental treatment, must be associated with dental hygiene education/motivation, as well as other topical fluorides if possible [10]. Besides that, the retentive cavities can be reshaped or partially opened with the use of manual instruments, aiming to remove the sites of plaque retention before SDF application and to facilitate the cleanability of the tooth and the disturbance of the dental plaque.

5. Evidence of silver diamine fluoride effects

The process of remineralization involves the replacement of minerals in partially demineralized enamel and dentin [30]. SDF is one of the fluoride-based treatments that has supporting evidence for its use for remineralization. In vitro, in situ, and ex vivo research design models make it possible to evaluate the mineral density, microhardness, lesion depth, and many other variables that reflect the remineralization effect both in enamel and dentin. Clinically, consistent reports of inactivated carious lesions in children are shown by a significant number of randomized clinical trials as well as systematic reviews and metanalysis.

5.1 Remineralizing effects in enamel

In vitro studies demonstrated that initial lesions in enamel can be remineralized with 38% SDF. In an artificial enamel caries model with bacterial pH challenge, the use of 38% SDF resulted in enhanced mineral density, with a higher depth of remineralization and better remineralization percentage when compared to the use of fluoride toothpaste alone [31]. The ability of remineralize early proximal enamel lesions was also demonstrated in an *in situ* study that showed similar increases in the mineral density after treatment with SDF and glass ionomer cement [32].

SDF was also effective in preventing demineralization. The demineralization inhibition effect of SDF treatment is mainly associated with the F2 in SDF [26]. When SDF is applied in sound enamel blocks and these blocks are artificially demineralized, SDF prevented the development of the enamel carious lesions when compared to $AgNO_3$ or KF [33]. After pH cycling, the SDF treated enamel remained with a relatively dense surface when compared to the use of NaF alone, with a higher content of fluoride and mineral density values and decreased lesion depths [34].

5.2 SDF in dentin

Dentin remineralization after SDF application promoted an outer layer of high mineralized dentine (approximately 150 μ), with a considerable presence of calcium and phosphate [23]. As a consequence of the remineralization, dentin carious lesions treated with 38% SDF also showed enhanced microhardness, which can be used as an indirect way (or a surrogate outcome in research) to identify changes in the mineral content of mineralized tissue. This was shown in an ex vivo study, where primary upper anterior teeth with dentin carious lesions received 38% SDF (one application every 12 months) [35].

Besides surface mineralization which is related to increased hardness, functional mineralization is also obtained; both characteristics can be achieved with the use of 38% SDF and are related to the mineral content of the tooth [36].

There are also important changes in the collagen fiber network. While in carious dentin, the collagen fibers are exposed due to demineralization, after 38% SDF application, the mineral loss and collagen exposure are reduced and a dense granular structure of spherical grains on the surface of the demineralized dentin is seen in artificial carious dentin treated with SDF under SEM [37]. It was also shown, in extracted teeth with carious lesions, that the collagen fiber network is protected with mineral after SDF treatment and the hydroxyapatite crystals exhibited a

Authors, year of publication	Number of included RCT/ number of patients	Objective	Main findings
Rosenblatt et al., 2009	2/827	To evaluate the effectiveness of silver diamine fluoride (SDF) to prevent caries when compared to fluoride varnish	SDF is more effective than fluoride varnish and may be a valuable caries-preventive intervention
Duangthip et al., 2015	4/967	To assess the effectiveness of non-surgical treatments of dentin caries in primary teeth in preschool children	SDF applications once/twice a year and daily toothbrushing with fluoride toothpaste appear to arrest or slow down the progression of active dentin caries in primary teeth in preschool children, but there is limited evidence to support this finding
Gao et al., 2016a	17/not reported	To investigate the clinical efficacy of professional fluoride therapy in remineralizing and arresting caries in children	Professionally applied 5% sodium fluoride varnish can remineralize early enamel caries and 38% silver diamine fluoride is effective in arresting dentine caries
Gao et al., 2016b	19/not reported	To investigate the clinical effectiveness of silver diamine fluoride (SDF) in arresting dental caries among children	38% SDF was effective in arresting dentin caries in primary teeth among children. The overall percentage of active caries that became arrested was 81%
Chibinski et al., 2017	11/4328	To evaluate the efficacy of silver diamine fluoride (SDF) in controlling caries progression in children when compared with active treatments or placebos	The use of SDF is 89% more effective in controlling/arresting caries than other treatments or placebo
Contreras et al., 2017	7/not reported	To evaluate the scientific evidence regarding the effectiveness of silver diamine fluoride (SDF) in preventing and arresting caries in the primary dentition and permanent first molars	SDF is a preventive treatment for dental caries in community settings. At concentrations of 30 and 38%, SDF shows potential as an alternative treatment for caries arrest in the primary dentition and permanent first molars
Oliveira et al., 2019	4/not reported	To investigate whether silver diamine fluoride (SDF) is effective in preventing new caries lesions in primary teeth when compared to placebo or active treatments	When applied to caries lesions in primary teeth, SDF compared to no treatment, placebo or fluoride varnish appears to effectively prevent dental caries in the entire dentition. However, trials specifically designed to assess this outcome are needed
Trieu et al., 2019	4/746	To evaluate the dentine caries arrest capabilities of silver diamine fluoride (SDF) and sodium fluoride (NaF).	SDF is a more effective caries management reagent than NaF (fluoride varnish)

Table 2.
Systematic reviews and meta-analysis that evaluated the effectiveness of SDF use in primary teeth.

well-aligned deposition. These favorable characteristics of the carious dentin were observed in an ex vivo study that analyzed exfoliated teeth 24 months after SDF treatment [23].

5.3 Clinical SDF effectiveness: systematic reviews and meta-analysis

For this book chapter, it was chosen to describe the effectiveness of SDF based on systematic reviews and meta-analysis about SDF use/effectiveness in children.

Systematic reviews (SR) and meta-analysis (MA) can be seen as a magnifying glass [38] from which the available evidence is evaluated. In applying a rigorous and methodic way to collect and analyze the data, systematic reviews and meta-analysis group the evidence and facilitate the decision-making process for stakeholders and clinicians. Therefore, the use of SR and MA eliminates the need of analyzing individual randomized clinical trials, while providing a broad and rigorous process of study selection and a statistical analysis of the data retrieved from all the papers that fulfill the quality control established by the authors.

The set of systematic reviews and meta-analysis about SDF are listed in **Table 2**. From the eight available papers, three are systematic reviews without meta-analysis [6, 39, 40]; and two did not evaluate SDF specifically, but as part of professionally applied fluoride treatments [41] and non-surgical treatments for caries arrestment [39].

Although different SR and MA establish distinct approaches to treat data, especially regarding the inclusion of high risk of bias papers in the metanalysis [41, 42] and the lack of overall quality of the evidence evaluation (GRADE) [6, 19, 39–43], all the papers concluded that SDF is superior to other tested strategies when caries arrestment is considered. SDF was found to be more effective than fluoride varnish [6, 22, 44], atraumatic restorative treatment [22] or placebo treatments [22].

The possibility of SDF application offering protection to all the deciduous dentition from the patient that received SDF treatment was analyzed by one of the RS and MA [43]. Despite the reduced number of included studies, the authors pointed out that it seems to be a protector effect after SDF use, since it decreased the number of new lesions in 77%, which shows that maybe SDF can be able to prevent the development of carious lesions in all deciduous dentition.

Finally, an umbrella review has been published in 2019 [45]. This type of study can be considered an overview of systematic reviews and aimed to provide a low-bias, comprehensive assessment of the evidence from the available systematic reviews related to the use of SDF for the management of carious lesions in children and adults. This paper concluded that the effectiveness of SDF for arresting coronal caries in deciduous dentition is a consistent finding among all the systematic reviews evaluated and the available evidence is strong. Therefore, the pediatric dentist can be very confident when using SDF in his/her daily practice, since this non-invasive treatment has a strong history of evidence behind it.

6. How silver diamine fluoride is applied?

6.1 What is important to know before clinical treatment with SDF?

The use of SDF preserves all dental tissue. Therefore, total or selective carious tissue removal is not needed.

Accidental contact of SDF with patient's or practitioner's skin can cause a brown stain that will be eliminated within 2–14 days due to natural exfoliation of the dead outer skin tissues. A brown stain will be permanent if there is accidental contact of SDF with clothes and other surfaces of dental clinic not protect by a barrier like a plastic liner [46].

SDF is an alkaline solution, if inadvertent contact with gingival tissue or mucosa occurs, reversible localized changes, represented by small and mildly pain white lesions or transient gingivitis, will appear [47]. These lesions disappear in 48 h, without any treatment [26]. Therefore, it is recommended to cover soft tissues nearby the site of SDF application, as well as lips and skin around the mouth, with petroleum jelly to prevent accidental contact.

Informed consent must be obtained from parents before SDF treatment. The informed consent form should describe all the benefits and side-effects related to the use of SDF, including the fact that SDF is not a restorative procedure, but a very effective anticaries agent. The dentist must provide all the needed information about the procedure in a simple and clear language, aiming for an easy understanding of the parents. At this moment, additional resources like pictures of teeth treated with SDF can be used to aid the professional in explaining the treatment. Photos showing the appearance of teeth before and after SDF application are a valuable resource to describe the darkening of the teeth; at the same time, the parents must be ensured that sound enamel will not be stained.

6.2 Application technique

The first step is the selection of the material needed for the SDF application: toothbrush, petroleum jelly, glass Dappen dish, disposable applicators, cotton rolls, and SDF solution (**Figure 2**). If the application is done in the dental office, the toothbrush is not needed, since dental prophylaxis with Robinson brush can be done.

The application technique of the SDF is a very simple procedure and is exemplified in **Figures 3–6**. The steps involved are described below [48]:

- Dental prophylaxis: the biofilm must be removed from the dental surface (enamel or dentin). For this purpose, the professional may use toothbrush, wet cotton pellets or, if dental office is available, a dental prophylaxis with Robinson brush and pumice/water paste;

- Soft tissues must be protected with petroleum jelly, including lips, gums, and perioral soft tissues to avoid direct contact with SDF solution;

- The operation field must be isolated with cotton rolls;

- Before dispensing a drop of SDF solution in a glass Dappen dish, the solution must be agitated for homogenization;

- The tooth surface or cavity that will receive the SDF treatment must be dried with dry cotton pellets or a gentle flow of compressed air;

- SDF solution must be actively applied with disposable tips; application time should be about 1 minute;

- A gentle flow of compressed air can be applied to help the solution to dry; during this process, the isolation of the operatory field must be on place;

- After approximately 3 minutes, if possible, the isolation can be removed.

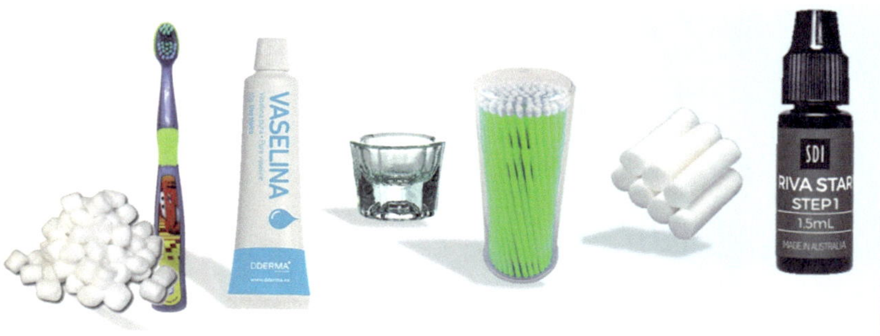

Figure 2.
Material used for a SDF treatment.

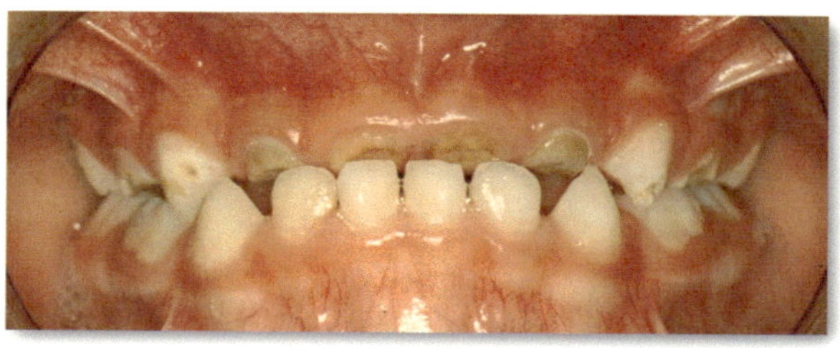

Figure 3.
Patient with early childhood caries, exhibiting active caries lesions in enamel and dentin.

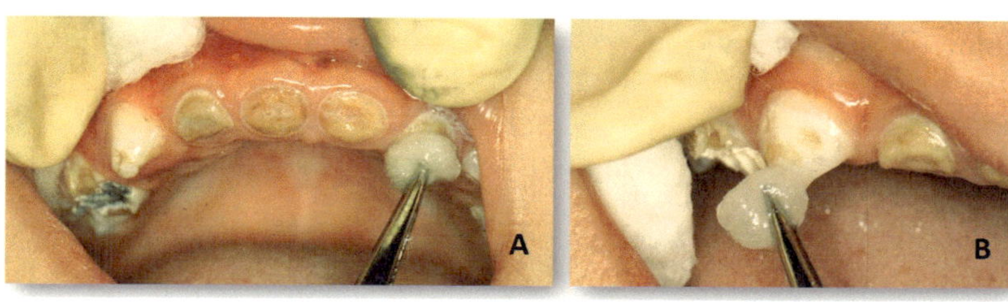

Figure 4.
*(A and B) SDF application was done in all active lesions, including upper anterior teeth (**Figure 4A**) and enamel lesions (**Figure 4B**). This procedure was taken to paralyze the progression of carious lesions during the modification of dietary and oral hygiene habits. Operative treatment was done afterward in specific teeth.*

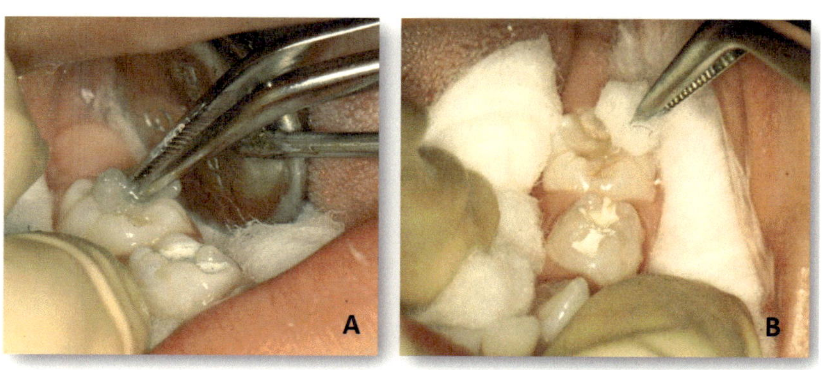

Figure 5.
(A and B) SDF was also applied on occlusal surfaces of deciduous primary molars.

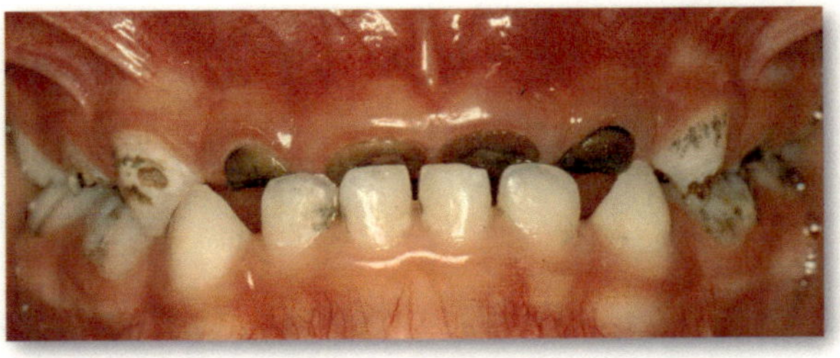

Figure 6.
Clinical aspect in a follow-up consultation: darkening is evident without the progress of the carious lesions.

The application times can be shortened without any prejudice for the cariostatic effect when treating very young or very difficult to manage patients. Notwithstanding, the professional must monitor carefully at post-op consultation the lesion appearance; if it does not exhibit a darker and harder surface, re-application is needed.

6.3 Tooth staining: how do parents, patients, and dentists deal with?

Tooth staining is the main adverse effect related to the SDF application. It is related to the formation of metallic silver from silver compounds [19]. As a result, all carious tissue – enamel and dentin – will become dark brown or black in a short period after SDF application and this may be an obstacle to SDF usage.

The dental literature shows that distinct factors can influence the parent's acceptance. Between these factors included the type of tooth (anterior or posterior), family income, parental schooling, ethnicity, and need for advanced behavior control methods [49].

Parents of uncooperative children tend to better accept the tooth staining to avoid more advanced behavior guidance, like sedation or general anesthesia [49–51].

The possibility of pain-free treatment is considered the most important factor when choosing a treatment by 74% of the parents; esthetics were considered the main goal only by 26% of the parents [51]. It is also common the statement that the staining would not be of major concern if the dental problem of the children can be solved [52, 53]. Notwithstanding, these results came from studies developed in Saudi Arabia [51] and Brazil [52, 53] and may not reflect the reality in other countries.

Anyway, the SDF application is better accepted in posterior compared to anterior teeth [10, 50, 51] and in deciduous compared to permanent teeth [51].

There is a trend toward high-income parents to choose esthetics. Parents with high or middle income and with a higher educational level are less likely to accept the use of SDF and the staining [10, 49].

Regarding professionals, a prejudice toward SDF staining may prevent a broader use or even make it difficult for them to offer this treatment to patients and parents [49]. In other words, dentists may assume that parents will not accept SDF treatment, with a preconception that esthetic is their main concern [49].

Therefore, it is important for the professional to fully understand the advantages and disadvantages of SDF treatment and the clinical situations that SDF can be a valuable resource. At the same time, the parent's and patient's opinions must be taken into account when deciding a treatment plan for a child. This should be done after a conversation about all the available treatment methods, considering not only the dentist's personal preferences but mainly the needs and wishes of the patient and his/her parents.

6.4 Tooth staining: is potassium iodide (KI) the answer?

The use of potassium iodide (KI) after SDF application has been proposed as an alternative to eliminate or minimize the tooth staining [54]. Currently, there is only one product that presents this association (Riva Star – SDI, Australia).

Silver phosphate is the subproduct of the SDF reaction with hydroxyapatite that is the main responsible for the tooth staining. If a saturated solution of KI (1 g KI/mL) is applied after SDF treatment, the subsequent reaction will result in silver iodide (AgI) and tripotassium phosphate (K_3PO_4). The last one is the chemical substance responsible for the reduction of tooth staining, while silver iodide can still promote some staining because it is a photosensitive subproduct [55].

The protocol of the SDF application is as follows:

- after application of SDF, keep the relative isolation in position and remove the excess of the SDF solution with a gauze or a cotton roll;
- KI solution must be applied to the tooth with a new disposable applicator;
- at this point, the solution will become creamy white; this is due to the formation of tripotassium phosphate;
- the application of KI solution should be repeated for 2 or 3 times, with a 5–10 s interval between applications, until no more white precipitates can be seen;
- the excess of the KI solution must be removed with gauze or cotton roll;
- the tooth is washed with water and the relative isolation can be removed.

So far, there are no randomized clinical trials that evaluate the effect of the association of SDF with KI. A systematic review of in vitro studies that evaluated the reduction of tooth staining after the SDF + KI application concluded that there seems to exist a positive effect in this association. However, since the methodologies of the studies are very different, direct comparisons are difficult and this conclusion must be validated by future well-designed studies [56].

7. How is the deciduous pulp reaction to the SDF application?

The possibility of an increased incidence of pulp lesions associated with the SDF application is not supported by data from randomized clinical trials [56, 57].

This finding is corroborated by histological studies, which showed that carious deciduous dentin treated with 38% SDF exhibited hypermineralization of the intertubular dentin [58], with a higher content of calcium and phosphorus [59] and a few blocked tubules [58]. Beneath that hypermineralized region, the tubules had characteristics of normality.

At the pulp area associated with the carious lesion, chronic inflammatory infiltrate could be seen [58], which did not halt the formation of tertiary dentin [58, 60]. This apposition of minerals in the intra and intertubular dentin after an exogenous stimulus is representative of a tooth with a vital pulpo-dentinal organ [23]. The odontoblastic layer may be flattened, but without further histological changes [60].

Silver deposits are more commonly seen along dentinal tubules than in the body of dentin. The silver penetration is facilitated by the demineralization of enamel and dentin and it can reach dental pulp tissue in deep cavities [59].

The literature is very limited on this topic and the data described in this chapter is based on ex vivo studies with very small samples, on which deciduous teeth that received 38% SDF application 6–12 months before exfoliation were collected and studied [58, 60]. Therefore, the findings, despite encouraging, should be considered preliminary and new studies are needed to further clarify this topic.

8. Conclusion

SDF is a non-invasive, painless, and effective treatment for the management of carious lesions in children. Considering the simplicity and safety of its use, it is a strategy that can be applied in individual or collective levels and can be associated with other non-invasive, micro-invasive or minimally invasive strategies.

The use of SDF fulfills the World Health Organization (WHO) Millennium Development Goals for Health and can contribute to the reduction of the inequities in oral health around the globe as well as provide a friendly treatment approach in Pediatric Dentistry daily clinic.

Acknowledgements

The author thanks Prof. Denise Stadler Wambier for the concession of the clinical photos used to illustrate this chapter.

Conflict of interest

The author declares no conflict of interest.

Author details

Ana Cláudia Rodrigues Chibinski*
State University of Ponta Grossa, Ponta Grossa, Brazil

*Address all correspondence to: anachibinski@uepg.br

References

[1] Peres MA, Macpherson LMD, Weyant RJ, Daly B, Venturelli R, Mathur MR, et al. Oral diseases: A global public health challenge. The Lancet. 2019;**394**:249-260. DOI: 10.1016/s0140-6736(19)31146-8

[2] Kassebaum NJ, Smith AGC, Bernabé E, Fleming TD, Reynolds AE, Vos T, et al. Global, regional, and national prevalence, incidence, and disability-adjusted life years for Oral conditions for 195 countries, 1990-2015: A systematic analysis for the global burden of diseases, injuries, and risk factors. Journal of Dental Research. 2017;**96**:380-387. DOI: 10.1177/0022034517693566

[3] Machiulskiene V, Campus G, Carvalho JC, Dige I, Ekstrand KR, Jablonski-Momeni A, et al. Terminology of dental caries and dental caries management: Consensus report of a workshop organized by ORCA and cardiology research group of IADR. Caries Research. 2020;**54**:7-14. DOI: 10.1159/000503309

[4] Frencken JE. Atraumatic restorative treatment and minimal intervention dentistry. British Dental Journal. 2017;**223**:183-189. DOI: 10.1038/sj.bdj.2017.664

[5] Schwendicke F, Splieth C, Breschi L, Banerjee A, Fontana M, Paris S, et al. When to intervene in the caries process? An expert Delphi consensus statement. Clinical Oral Investigations. 2019;**23**:3691-3703. DOI: 10.1007/s00784-019-03058-w

[6] Rosenblatt A, Stamford T, Niederman R. Silver diamine fluoride: A caries "silver-fluoride bullet". Journal of Dental Research. 2009;**88**:116-125

[7] Crystal YO, Marghalani AA, Ureles SD, Wright JT, Sulyanto R, Divaris K, et al. Use of silver diamine fluoride for dental caries management in children and adolescents, including those with special health care needs. Pediatric Dentistry. 2017;**39**:135-145

[8] Zhao IS, Gao SS, Hiraishi N, Burrow MF, Duangthip D, Mei ML, et al. Mechanisms of silver diamine fluoride on arresting caries: A literature review. International Dental Journal. 2018;**68**:67-76

[9] Duangthip D, Chu C, Lo E. A randomized clinical trial on arresting dentine caries in preschool children by topical fluorides—18 month results. Journal of Dentistry. 2016;**44**:57-63

[10] Fung M, Duangthip D, Wong M, Lo E, Chu C. Randomized clinical trial of 12% and 38% silver diamine fluoride treatment. Journal of Dental Research. 2018;**97**:171-178

[11] Milgrom P, Horst JA, Ludwig S, Rothen M, Chaffee BW, Lyalina S, et al. Topical silver diamine fluoride for dental caries arrest in preschool children: A randomized controlled trial and microbiological analysis of caries associated microbes and resistance gene expression. Journal of Dentistry. 2018;**68**:72-78

[12] Yee R, Holmgren C, Mulder J, Lama D, Walker D, van Palenstein Helderman W. Efficacy of silver diamine fluoride for arresting caries treatment. Journal of Dental Research. 2009;**88**:644-647

[13] Zhi QH, Lo ECM, Lin HC. Randomized clinical trial on effectiveness of silver diamine fluoride and glass ionomer in arresting dentine caries in preschool children. Journal of Dentistry. 2012;**40**:962-967

[14] Braga M, Mendes F, De Benedetto M, Imparato J. Effect of silver diammine fluoride on incipient

caries lesions in erupting permanent first molars: A pilot study. Journal of Dentistry for Children. 2009;**76**:28-33

[15] Liu B, Lo E, Chu C, Lin H. Randomized trial on fluorides and sealants for fissure caries prevention. Journal of Dental Research. 2012;**91**:753-758

[16] Timms L, Sumner O, Deery C, Rogers HJ. Everyone else is using it, so why isn't the UK? Silver diamine fluoride for children and young people. Community Dental Health. 2020;**37**:143-149. DOI: 10.1922/CDH_00008Timms07

[17] Zander V, Chan D, Sadr A. Microcomputed tomography evaluation of root dentin caries prevention by topical fluorides and potassium iodide. Sensors. 2019;**19**:874

[18] Hu S, Meyer B, Duggal M. A silver renaissance in dentistry. European Archives of Paediatric Dentistry. 2018;**19**:221-227

[19] Peng JJ, Botelho MG, Matinlinna JP. Silver compounds used in dentistry for caries management: A review. Journal of Dentistry. 2012;**40**:531-541. DOI: 10.1016/j.jdent.2012.03.009

[20] Mei M, Lo E, Chu C. Arresting dentine caries with silver diamine fluoride: what's behind it? Journal of Dental Research. 2018;**97**:751-758

[21] Yu OY, Zhao IS, Mei ML, Lo ECM, Chu CH. Caries-arresting effects of silver diamine fluoride and sodium fluoride on dentine caries lesions. Journal of Dentistry. 2018;**78**:65-71. DOI: 10.1016/j.jdent.2018.08.007

[22] Chibinski AC, Wambier LM, Feltrin J, Loguercio AD, Wambier DS, Reis A. Silver diamine fluoride has efficacy in controlling caries progression in primary teeth: A systematic review and meta-analysis. Caries Research. 2017;**51**:527-541

[23] Mei ML, Ito L, Cao Y, Lo EC, Li Q, Chu C. An ex vivo study of arrested primary teeth caries with silver diamine fluoride therapy. Journal of Dentistry. 2014;**42**:395-402

[24] Seifo N, Robertson M, MacLean J, Blain K, Grosse S, Milne R, et al. The use of silver diamine fluoride (SDF) in dental practice. British Dental Journal. 2020;**228**:75-81

[25] Crystal YO, Niederman R. Evidence-based dentistry update on silver Diamine fluoride. Dental Clinics. 2019;**63**:45-68

[26] Horst JA, Ellenikiotis H, Milgrom PL. UCSF protocol for caries arrest using silver diamine fluoride: Rationale, indications and consent. Journal of the California Dental Association. 2016;**44**:16-28

[27] Hammersmith KJ, DePalo JR, Casamassimo PS, MacLean JK, Peng J. Silver diamine fluoride and fluoride varnish may halt interproximal caries progression in the primary dentition. The Journal of Clinical Pediatric Dentistry. 2020;**44**:79-83. DOI: 10.17796/1053-4625-44.2.2

[28] Fung M, Duangthip D, Wong M, Lo E, Chu C. Arresting dentine caries with different concentration and periodicity of silver diamine fluoride. JDR Clinical & Translational Research. 2016;**1**:143-152

[29] Huang W-T, Shahid S, Anderson P. Applications of silver diamine fluoride in management of dental caries. In: Khurshid Z, Najeeb S, Zafar MS, Sefat F, editors. Advanced Dental Biomaterials. Cambridge, United Kingdom: Elsevier; 2019. pp. 675-699

[30] González-Cabezas C, Fernández CE. Recent advances

in remineralization therapies for caries lesions. Advances in Dental Research. 2018;**29**:55-59. DOI: 10.1177/0022034517740124

[31] Punyanirun K, Yospiboonwong T, Kunapinun T, Thanyasrisung P, Trairatvorakul C. Silver diamine fluoride remineralized artificial incipient caries in permanent teeth after bacterial pH-cycling in-vitro. Journal of Dentistry. 2018;**69**:55-59

[32] Nantanee R, Santiwong B, Trairatvorakul C, Hamba H, Tagami J. Silver diamine fluoride and glass ionomer differentially remineralize early caries lesions, in situ. Clinical Oral Investigations. 2016;**20**:1151-1157. DOI: 10.1007/s00784-015-1603-4

[33] Sorkhdini P, Gregory RL, Crystal YO, Tang Q, Lippert F. Effectiveness of in vitro primary coronal caries prevention with silver diamine fluoride - chemical vs biofilm models. Journal of Dentistry. 2020. Article ID: 103418. DOI: 10.1016/j.jdent.2020.103418

[34] Yu OY, Mei ML, Zhao IS, Li Q-L, Lo EC-M, Chu C-H. Remineralisation of enamel with silver diamine fluoride and sodium fluoride. Dental Materials. 2018;**34**:e344-ee52

[35] Chu CH, Lo EC. Microhardness of dentine in primary teeth after topical fluoride applications. Journal of Dentistry. 2008;**36**:387-391. DOI: 10.1016/j.jdent.2008.02.013

[36] Firouzmandi M, Shafiei F, Jowkar Z, Nazemi F. Effect of silver diamine fluoride and proanthocyanidin on mechanical properties of caries-affected dentin. European Journal of Dentistry. 2019;**13**:255-260. DOI: 10.1055/s-0039-1693237

[37] Mei ML, Ito L, Cao Y, Li Q, Lo EC, Chu C. Inhibitory effect of silver diamine fluoride on dentine demineralisation and collagen degradation. Journal of Dentistry. 2013;**41**:809-817

[38] Murad MH, Asi N, Alsawas M, Alahdab F. New evidence pyramid. Evidence-Based Medicine. 2016;**21**: 125-127. DOI: 10.1136/ebmed-2016-110401

[39] Duangthip D, Jiang M, Chu CH, Lo EC. Non-surgical treatment of dentin caries in preschool children--systematic review. BMC Oral Health. 2015;**15**:44. DOI: 10.1186/s12903-015-0033-7

[40] Contreras V, Toro MJ, Elías-Boneta AR, Encarnación-Burgos A. Effectiveness of silver diamine fluoride in caries prevention and arrest: A systematic literature review. General Dentistry. 2017;**65**:22-29

[41] Gao SS, Zhang S, Mei ML, Lo EC-M, Chu C-H. Caries remineralisation and arresting effect in children by professionally applied fluoride treatment–a systematic review. BMC Oral Health. 2016;**16**:12

[42] Gao S, Zhao I, Hiraishi N, Duangthip D, Mei M, Lo E, et al. Clinical trials of silver diamine fluoride in arresting caries among children: A systematic review. JDR Clinical & Translational Research. 2016;**1**(3):201-210

[43] Oliveira BH, Rajendra A, Veitz-Keenan A, Niederman R. The effect of silver diamine fluoride in preventing caries in the primary dentition: A systematic review and meta-analysis. Caries Research. 2019;**53**:24-32

[44] Trieu A, Mohamed A, Lynch E. Silver diamine fluoride versus sodium fluoride for arresting dentine caries in children: A systematic review and meta-analysis. Scientific Reports. 2019;**9**:1-9

[45] Seifo N, Cassie H, Radford JR, Innes NP. Silver diamine fluoride for

managing carious lesions: An umbrella review. BMC Oral Health. 2019;**19**:145

[46] Horst J. Silver fluoride as a treatment for dental caries. Advances in Dental Research. 2018;**29**:135-140

[47] Mei ML, Lo EC, Chu CH. Clinical use of silver diamine fluoride in dental treatment. Compendium of Continuing Education in Dentistry. 2016;**37**:93-98

[48] Guide C. Silver diamine fluoride in the management of dental caries lesions. Pediatric Dentistry. 2018;**40**:492-517

[49] Magno MB, Silva LPD, Ferreira DM, Barja-Fidalgo F, Fonseca-Gonçalves A. Aesthetic perception, acceptability and satisfaction in the treatment of caries lesions with silver diamine fluoride: A scoping review. International Journal of Paediatric Dentistry. 2019;**29**:257-266. DOI: 10.1111/ipd.12465

[50] Crystal Y, Kreider B, Raveis V. Parental expressed concerns about silver diamine fluoride (SDF) treatment. The Journal of Clinical Pediatric Dentistry. 2019;**43**:155-160

[51] Bagher SM, Sabbagh HJ, AlJohani SM, Alharbi G, Aldajani M, Elkhodary H. Parental acceptance of the utilization of silver diamine fluoride on their child's primary and permanent teeth. Patient Preference and Adherence. 2019;**13**:829

[52] Triches TC, Cordeiro MMR, Souza JGMV, Saltori EK, França BHS. Aceitação dos pais quanto ao uso do diaminofluoreto de prata em crianças de 0 a 3 anos de Cascavel/PR. Pesquisa Brasileira em Odontopediatria e Clínica Integrada. 2009;**9**:265-269

[53] Belotti L, Citty LS, Gomes AMM. A Aplicabilidade do diaminofluoreto de Prata em Crianças de 4 a 10 anos de Idade na Clínica de Odontopediatria da Universidade Federal do Espírito Santo, Brasil. Journal of Health Sciences. 2016;**18**:5-12

[54] Patel J, Anthonappa RP, King NM. Evaluation of the staining potential of silver diamine fluoride: In vitro. International Journal of Paediatric Dentistry. 2018;**28**:514-522

[55] Garg S, Sadr A, Chan D. Potassium iodide reversal of silver diamine fluoride staining: A case report. Operative Dentistry. 2019;**44**:221-226

[56] Chu C, Lo E, Lin H. Effectiveness of silver diamine fluoride and sodium fluoride varnish in arresting dentin caries in Chinese pre-school children. Journal of Dental Research. 2002;**81**:767-770

[57] Llodra J, Rodriguez A, Ferrer B, Menardia V, Ramos T, Morato M. Efficacy of silver diamine fluoride for caries reduction in primary teeth and first permanent molars of schoolchildren: 36-month clinical trial. Journal of Dental Research. 2005;**84**:721-724

[58] Rossi G, Squassi A, Mandalunis P, Kaplan A. Effect of silver diamine fluoride (SDF) on the dentin-pulp complex: Ex vivo histological analysis on human primary teeth and rat molars. Acta Odontológica Latinoamericana. 2017;**30**:5-12

[59] Li Y, Liu Y, Psoter WJ, Nguyen OM, Bromage TG, Walters MA, et al. Assessment of the silver penetration and distribution in carious lesions of deciduous teeth treated with silver diamine fluoride. Caries Research. 2019;**53**:432-441

[60] Bimstein E, Damm D. Human primary tooth histology six months after treatment with silver diamine fluoride. The Journal of Clinical Pediatric Dentistry. 2018;**42**:442-444

Chapter 7

Caries Experience and Oral Disorders of Disabled Children

Berna Kuter

Abstract

Dental caries is a major health problem for disabled children. These special children have chronic diseases; oral disorders; and physical, mental, behavioral, and cognitive impairments; and sensual disorders. They have higher and more severe oral disorders than healthy children, and the majority of these children have poor oral hygiene with high caries prevalence and gingivitis. These special children suffer from oral disease, especially in terms of periodontal disease, oral mucosal pathology, and malocclusion. Parents and caregivers must be educated and encouraged regarding these special children's dental care and tooth brushing. The dentist should know more information about these special children and should be more careful during treatment. Pediatric dentists must take care of special attention to the oral healthcare of these special children and help them to have healthy smiles.

Keywords: dental caries, disabled children, oral health, oral disorders, oral hygiene

1. Introduction

Dental problems are more common among disabled children [1]. This situation is due to both mental disability and insufficient oral health care. Disabled children need special dental care [2]. They have chronic diseases, poor oral hygiene and physical, mental, behavioral, cognitive impairment and sensual disorders [2]. Furthermore, the articles reported that they had more untreated caries, poorer oral health, periodontitis and fewer remaining teeth [3, 4]. The disabled children could not understand and take responsibility for cooperate with preventive oral health practices [5]. Information about pain in these children is inadequate and less trustworthy for a physician [1, 2]. The dentist should know more knowledge about these special children and should be more careful during treatment [5]. Therefore, it is important to know data especially about the oral health of disabled children. First of all, it could be useful to learn about the oral hygiene and dental caries of disabled children to prevent their dental caries and provide good oral hygiene. Moreover, having more information about oral hygiene and dental caries status of these special children will provide an easier treatment process for both dentist and disabled children.

2. Dental caries and disabled children

A high caries value was declared among disabled children [6–8]. It was reported that the oral hygiene of disabled children was poor, and they need dental treatment [9, 10]. These children have problem in brushing their teeth [11].

IntechOpen

Pain is a subjective experience that to alert them of danger [12]. It limits exposure to additional injury. Children learn to preclude and overcome their pain. However, it is very difficult to define pain especially for disabled children [13]. Untreated, acute or chronic pain could have significant and lifelong consequences [12]. Pain, fear and anxiety are similar for children and they usually confound them. However, disabled children have a problem of not being able to clarify pain, in additionally [13]. Parents or caregivers usually describe that disabled children's pain, experience and treatment [14, 15]. It was stated that disabled children have more pain than the healthy individuals because of systemic diseases associated with their disorders. It is appeared to have more caries risk factors such as associated medical conditions and intake of medications in disabled children [16].

Oral disorder is significant health problem for disabled children [17]. They have a higher prevalence and severity of oral disease compared to the healthy children. Dental caries, missing teeth, supernumerary teeth prolonged retention of primary teeth, periodontal disease, crowding and malocclusion are causes poor oral health in these special children.

It was stated that the DMFT score of mentally disabled children was significantly higher, while the dft values of healthy children was higher [16]. Some researchers reported that the disabled children had higher both DMFT and dft indices compared to healthy children [18, 19]. These special children could be more susceptible to dental caries if they reside at home and feeding with cardiogenic snacks and other unhealthy foods [20]. It was reported that disabled children have more dental problems and more untreated dental disease relative to other children [18, 19].

3. Oral hygiene and disabled children

Disabled children often depend on parents and caregivers for oral hygiene practices in comparison with healthy children who take care of their own oral health [21]. It was stated that these special children suffered from dental disease up to seven times as frequently as the healthy children, particularly with respect to periodontal disease, oral mucosal pathology and malocclusion [22, 23].

Caregivers must be educated and encouraged regarding these special children' dental care and tooth brushing [24]. Dentists should also be encouraged regarding the proper training of parents and caregivers. Tesini stated regular contact should be provided with their families and caregivers and they should be educated on diet to improve oral hygiene [25].

Some researchers explained that the use of anticonvulsant medications that affect gum health [26, 27], parent and caregivers' poor understanding of the importance of dental hygiene and the fear of dental treatment [28] promoted poor oral health among disabled children.

4. A major cariogenic organism: *Streptococcus mutans* and disabled children

Streptococcus mutans was a major etiologic agent for dental caries [29]. It is a major cariogenic organism that contributes to the formation of dental biofilm matrix and produces large amounts of organic acids [30]. It was defined that a gene was as a DNA segment [31, 32]. It contributes to phenotype and genotype is the genetic structure of an organism or a cell. Children usually have fewer *S. mutans* genotype than adults and *S. mutans* genotype c is the most common form of dental caries in children [33].

It is important to evaluate and compare the variety of *S. mutans* genotypes with respect to caries activity among healthy and mentally disabled children and to plan better strategies for early caries detection, prevention and management [34]. It was found that genotype encoding Primer 1 was present 82.5% in total population of both groups (healthy and mentally disabled children) and genotype encoding Primer 2 was present in 95% of the total population. However, genotype encoding Primer 3 was present in 20% of children associated with healthy and mentally disabled children. Prabhakar et al. stated that there was a significant difference between healthy and mentally disabled children in the distribution of *S. mutans* genotypes, however, there was no significant difference between healthy and mentally disabled children regarding amount of *S. mutans*. Total of 52 distinct genotypes for healthy children were identified, however, mentally disabled children have fewer number of them [35].

It was found that *S. mutans* were available in Down syndrome children that were responsible for a low caries rate [36]. However, there is lack of evidence on the genotypic variety of *S. mutans* in the mentally disabled children and the relationship between its molecular diversity and the specific species of *S. mutans* that causes dental caries is yet to be understood [34].

5. Relationship between oral disorders and dental caries in the disabled children

Oral health of disabled children was worse than that of healthy children, because of the existing disability or social, economic or medical reasons [37]. Researches on the dental health of mentally disabled children showed that majority of the children had poor oral hygiene with high caries prevalence and gingivitis [38, 39]. Studies have also stated that disabled children have poor oral health and greater treatment needs than those of healthy children. Dental caries and the premature loss of primary teeth could lead to malocclusion in the permanent dentition [40]. Vellappally et al. stated that the prevalence of malocclusion and dental caries were found to be high in disabled children. However, it was reported that there was no positive correlation between caries and malocclusion in these children [41]. The other study [42] also revealed the same result in the mixed dentition. The results of the study revealed that the prevalence of malocclusion among mentally disabled children was 93%. Onyeaso reported 47% prevalence of malocclusion among mentally disabled children [43]. Furthermore, Baskaradoss et al. stated that a positive correlation was found between the dental caries and malocclusion and prevalence of malocclusion among mentally disabled children was much higher than that of healthy children [44]. Dental crowding, anterior diastema and antero-posterior molar relationship were reported as the common malocclusion among mentally disabled children by Dinesh et al. [45].

6. The most common types of disabled children with intra oral manifestations

6.1 Down syndrome

Down syndrome is an autosomal chromosomal disorder [46]. It is characterized by neurological changes, generalized hypotonia, structural cardiopathy, dental anomalies and orofacial dysmorphology [46–49]. The children with Down syndrome have specific orofacial features which include low prevalence of dental caries, macroglossia, fissured lips and tongue, microdontia, mouth breathing, open bite, delayed teeth eruption, missing and malformed teeth, crowding, malocclusion, posterior cross bite, abnormally rounded labial forms of the tooth crown, partial anodontia, periodontitis and bruxism [49].

The children with Down syndrome were more susceptible to periodontal disease, reduced levels of calculus and had a greater need for oral hygiene compared to those of healthy children was reported [24, 50]. Periodontal disease is the most significant oral health problem in these children [51]. The difficulties in tooth brushing and reduced manual dexterity could lead to poor oral hygiene in these children [21]. Barnett et al. investigated the prevalence rates of periodontitis and dental caries in children with Down syndrome [52]. When Down syndrome children and mentally disability children compared, results revealed a greater prevalence of periodontitis and a lower prevalence of dental caries in Down syndrome children. The literature revealed that differences in the composition of the microbiota, dental morphology and salivary composition in children with Down syndrome were led to the low prevalence of caries and higher prevalence of bruxism [53]. It was reported that some syndromes, which have chromosomal abnormalities to be associated with low caries indices, as in Down syndrome [54]. However, the reason of the low incidence of caries in Down syndrome is unclear.

Dental treatments of these patients are required special attention [47–49]. Porovic stated that Down syndrome children have a high prevalence of caries, and extraction as a treatment option [55]. It is important to create oral health care programs with parental education and it is necessary to educate dental practitioners to work with these children.

It was reported as an important risk factor for malocclusion [56], decreased arch length, reduced dental arch dimension and diminished maxillary size in Down syndrome children [56–58]. The studies have reported a high prevalence of anterior open bite, posterior crossbite and overjet in children with Down syndrome compared to other children [59].

6.2 Autism

Autism is defined by impaired functions of management, lack of attention, speech disorders, repetitive behaviors and communication difficulties [60]. Muhle reported that etiological factors causing autism were genetic, post-encephalitic infection, autoimmune factors and Vitamin D deficiency [61]. Autism is seen four times more in males than in females was reported [62]. The orthodontic disorders in autistic children are class II molar relationship, anterior open-bite, tongue thrusting and dental crowding [63]. Autistic children tend to keep food inside their mouths due to poor tongue coordination. Taking anticonvulsant drugs [64], unsuitable brushing habits, lack of communication, tend to keep it inside their mouths due to poor tongue coordination are caused of gingivitis and was stated that autistic children had more prevalence of caries degree than healthy children [65, 66]. However, the results of the other studies were reported no significant differences in the prevalence of caries degree, oral hygiene and gingivitis [67, 68]. On the contrary, some researchers reported that there is a lower incidence of dental caries in autistic children [39], and there was no statistically significant difference in periodontal health between the healthy and the autistic children [69]. Thus, it is seen that the articles were provided inconclusive answers concerning whether autism is a risk factor for caries and periodontal health.

It was reported that 26.4% of the autistic children had systemic diseases and 72.6% used medication [69]. Seventy-seven percent of autistic children used drugs were stated in the other study [70]. Specific drugs are prescribed for accompanying with autism such as hyperactivity, epilepsy and anxiety and the most common drugs taken by the autistic are antipsychotics, antidepressants and anticonvulsants [71]. It was thought that these drugs which used autistic children may be a reason of gingivitis because of their side effects. However, Marshall et al., stated that the psychoactive drugs have been not found to be a risk factor for caries in terms of xerostomia side effects [72].

It was reported that bruxism, tooth wear, deep-palate and tongue thrusting disorders were significantly higher percentage in the autistics than those of the healthy children [73]. Bruxism and tongue thrusting in the autistics could result in orthodontic disorders [74]. As a result, it was reported that the anterior open bite in autistics was significantly higher than that of the healthy in that study [70]. However, it was pronounced that no statistically significant differences were found between the autistics and healthy children related to the open bite in the other study [69]. Moreover, dental crowding in the healthy children was more than that of the autistic children in that study.

6.3 Cerebral palsy

Cerebral palsy is a common pediatric disorder resulting from a non-progressive deterioration to the developing brain and motor disorders are accompanied by disturbances in coordination, cognition, communication and seizure disorders [75, 76]. Muscle incompetence impairs lip seal and lead to an anterior posture of the tongue, an aberrant tongue and head posture, anterior crowding, anterior open bite, missing teeth, early eruption of primary teeth, anterior diastema [56, 77]. Class II malocclusions were most common features among children with cerebral palsy. It was also reported that a maxillary overjet in these children was reported to be the caused by lip deficiency and deformity of the maxillary orbicularis muscle. Studies have shown that these disorders lead to the higher risk of dental disease in these children [78]. Pseudo-bulbar palsy affects coordination of sucking, swallowing, chewing and excessive drooling which it could be related to increased production of saliva secondary to an irritating oral lesion, and dental caries [79]. Gastroesophageal reflux disease is common problem in children with cerebral palsy causing vomiting and it affects the dental health and results in dental erosions [80]. Dental erosion is common in these children and percentage of dental erosion is between 55% and 73% of cerebral palsy [81, 82]. It was stated that dental erosions affect both primary and permanent teeth, most commonly the upper molars, lower molars and upper incisors [83].

Motor incoordination affects the ability to perform adequate oral hygiene and as a result of this, gingival hyperplasia and associated bleeding occurs with higher frequency in children with cerebral palsy [84]. The use of antiepileptic drugs, particularly phenytoin is important factor for periodontal diseases.

Akhter et al. stated that children with cerebral palsy in a low-income had high dental caries experience [85].

Sialorrhea appears to be the consequence of a dysfunction in the coordination of swallowing mechanisms and occurs in up to 30% of children with cerebral palsy [79, 86].

It was reported that both bruxism and traumatic dental injuries were significantly higher percentage in children with cerebral palsy [77, 87]. The exact mechanisms causing the development of bruxism is not fully known, however, it was reported that it could be related to abnormal proprioception in the periodontium, sleep disorders could be predispose to the development of nocturnal bruxism, particularly in those with severe visual impairment [88].

Forty percent of children with cerebral palsy were born prematurely and they are at an increased risk for having developmental enamel defects and these defects are in a symmetrical manner in both primary incisors and first molars [89].

Children with cerebral palsy are at a significantly higher risk for developing temporomandibular joint disorders and boy gender, malocclusion, mouth breathing, and mixed dentition were identified as risk factors for developing this disorder [90].

7. Conclusions

It has been widely reported in literature that disabled children have poor oral healthcare and high caries prevalence. As the difficulties in tooth brushing and reduced manual dexterity could lead to dental caries and poor oral hygiene and these disabled children have a problem of not being able to clarify pain, it must be taken care of special attention in oral healthcare of these special children by dentists, their parents and caregivers.

Conflict of interest

No other relationships/conditions/circumstances that present a potential conflict of interest.

Author details

Berna Kuter
Faculty of Dentistry, Department of Paediatric Dentistry, Izmir Demokrasi University, Izmir, Turkey

*Address all correspondence to: berna.kuter@idu.edu.tr

References

[1] Kehitysvammalaki 519/1977. Law of intellectual disabilities. American Association on Intellectual and Developmental Disabilities (AAIDD); 2009. http://www.aaidd.org/content_100.cfm?navID=21. http://www.finlex.fi/fi/laki/alkup/1977/19770988

[2] Oredugba FA, Akindayomi Y. Oral health status and treatment needs of children and young adults attending a day centre for individuals with special health care needs. BMC Oral Health. 2008;**8**(30):1-8

[3] Nunn JH, Gordon PH, Carmichael CL. Dental disease and current treatment needs in a group of physically handicapped children. Community Dental Health Journal. 1993;**10**:389-396

[4] American Academy of Paediatric Dentistry Council on Clinical Affairs. Definition of persons with special health care needs [adopted 2004]. Pediatric Dentistry. 2005;**27**:15

[5] Bonito AJ. Executive summary: Dental care considerations for vulnerable populations. Special Care in Dentistry. 2002;**22**:5s-10s

[6] Alves NS, Gavina VP, Cortellazzi KL, Antunes LA, Silveira FM, Assaf AV. Analysis of clinical, demographic, socioeconomic, and psychosocial determinants of quality of life of persons with intellectual disability: A cross-sectional study. Special Care in Dentistry. 2016;**36**(6):307-314

[7] Abanto J, Carvalho TS, Bönecker M, Ortega AO, Ciamponi AL, Raggio DP. Parental reports of the oral health-related quality of life of children with cerebral palsy. BMC Oral Health. 2012;**12**(1):15

[8] Solanki J, Gupta S, Arya A. Dental caries and periodontal status of mentally handicapped institutilized children. Journal of Clinical and Diagnostic Research. 2014;**8**(7):25-27

[9] Faulks D, Norderyd J, Molina G, Macgiolla Phadraig C, Scagnet G, Eschevins C, et al. Using the international classification of functioning, disability and health (ICF) to describe children referred to special care or paediatric dental services. PLoS One. 2013;**8**(4):e61993, 1-12

[10] Aggarwal VP, Mathur A, Dileep CL, Batra M, Makkar DK. Impact of sociodemographic attributes and dental caries on quality of life of intellectual disabled children using ECOHIS. International Journal of Health Sciences (Qassim). 2016;**10**(4):480-490

[11] Shanmugam M, Shivakumar V, Anitha V, Meenapriya BP, Aishwarya S, Anitha R. Behavioral pattern during dental pain in intellectually disabled children: A comparative study. International Scholarly Research Notices. 2014;**18**:1-5

[12] Merskey H, Bogduk N. Classification of Chronic Pain: Description of Chronic Pain Syndromes and Definitions of Pain Terms. 2nd ed. Seattle, Washington, USA: IASP Press; 1994

[13] Franck LS, Greenberg CS, Stevens B. Pain assessment in infants and children. Pediatric Clinics of North America. 2000;**47**(3):487-512

[14] Stallard P, Williams L, Lenton S, Velleman R. Pain in cognitively impaired, non-communicating children. Archives of Disease in Childhood. 2001;**85**(6):460-462

[15] Fanurik D, Koh JL, Schmitz ML, Harrison RD, Conrad TM. Children with cognitive impairment: Parent report of pain and coping. Journal of Developmental & Behavioral Pediatrics. 1999;**20**(4):228-234

[16] Alaki SM, Bakry NS. Dental pain in children with intellectual disabilities: caregivers' perspective. International Journal of Dentistry. 2012;**2012**:7

[17] Altun C, Guven G, Akgun OM, Akkurt MD, Basak F, Akbulut E. Oral health Stastus of disabled individuals attending special schools. European Journal of Dentistry. 2010;**4**(4):361-366

[18] Reid BC, Chenette R, Macek MD. Prevalence and predictors of untreated caries and oral pain among Special Olympics athletes. Special Care in Dentistry. 2003;**23**:139-142

[19] Lewis C, Robertson AS, Phelps S. Unmet dental care needs among children with special health care needs: Implications for the medical home. Paediatrics. 2005;**116**:426-431

[20] White JA, Beltran ED, Malvitz DM, Perlman SP. Oral health status of special athletes in the San Francisco Bay area. Journal of the California Dental Association. 1998;**26**:347-354

[21] Kadam NS, Patil R, Gurav AN, Patil Y, Shete A, Naik Tari R, et al. Oral hygiene status, periodontal status, and periodontal treatment needs among institutionalized intellectually disabled subjects in Kolhapur District, Maharashtra, India. Journal of Oral Diseases. 2014. p. 1-11

[22] Anders PL, Davis EL. Oral health of patients with intellectual disabilities: A systematic review. Special Care in Dentistry. 2010;**30**:110-117

[23] Morgan JP, Minihan PM, Stark PC, Finkelman MD, Yantsides KE, Park A, et al. The oral health status of 4,732 adults with intellectual and developmental disabilities. Journal of the American Dental Association (1939). 2012;**143**:838-846

[24] Van Houtem C, De Jongh A, Broers D, Van Der Schoof M, Resida G. Post-academic specialties 9. Dental care of disabled children living at home. Ned Tijdschr Tandheelkd. 2007;**114**:129-133

[25] Tesini DA. An annotated review of the literature of dental caries and periodontal disease in mentally and physically retarded individuals. Special Care in Dentistry. 1981;**1**:75-87

[26] Siqueira WL, Santos MT, Elangovan S, Simoes A, Nicolau J. The influence of valproic acid on salivary pH in children with cerebral palsy. Special Care in Dentistry. 2007;**27**:64-66

[27] Sinha N, Singh B, Chhabra KG, Patil S. Comparison of oral health status between children with cerebral palsy and normal children in India: A case–control study. Journal of Indian Society of Periodontology. 2015;**19**:78-82

[28] Gordon SM, Dionne RA, Snyder J. Dental fear and anxiety as a barrier to accessing oral health care among patients with special health care needs. Special Care in Dentistry. 1998;**18**:88-92

[29] Loesche WJ. Role of *Streptococcus mutans* in human dental decay. Microbiological Reviews. 1986;**50**(4):353-380

[30] Banas JA, Vickerman MM. Glucan-binding proteins of the oral *Streptococci*. Critical Reviews in Oral Biology and Medicine. 2003;**14**(2):89-99

[31] Gerstein MB. What is a gene, post-encode? History and updated definition. Genome Research. 2007;**17**(6):669-681

[32] Arévalo-Ruano ML. Molecular identification and genotyping of *Streptococcus mutans* from saliva samples of children in Medellin, Colombia. CES Odontología. 2014;**27**(2):47-60

[33] KyoungaC,StephenAM,HowardWW, JenniferW, StephanieSM. Characteristics of *streptococcus mutans* genotypes and dental caries in children.

European Journal of Oral Sciences. 2013;**121**(301):148-155

[34] Prabhakar AR, Sreeja G, Naik SV. DNA finger printing of *S. mutans* present in the saliva of caries active children and those associated with intellectual disability—A RAPD analysis. Saudi Dental Journal. 2019;**31**(4):424-430

[35] Klein MI. Longitudinal study of transmission diversity, and stability of *Streptococcus mutans* and *Streptococcus sorbrinus* genotypes in Brazilian nursery children. Journal of Clinical Microbiology. 2004;**42**(10):4620-4626

[36] Cogulu D, Sabah E, Uzel A, Ozkinay F. Genotyping of *Streptococcus mutans* by using arbitrarily primed polymerase chain reaction in children with Down syndrome. Archives of Oral Biology. 2006;**51**(3):177-182

[37] Weng RH, Kung PT, Tsai WC, Chiang HH, Chiu LT. The use of fluoride varnish and its determining factors among children with disability in Taiwan. Research in Developmental Disabilities. 2011;**32**(2):583-592

[38] Saravanakumar M, Vasanthakumari A, Bharathan R. Oral health status of special health care needs children attending a day care centre in Chennai. International Journal of Students' Research. 2013;**3**(1):12

[39] Namal N, Vehit HE, Koksal S. Do autistic children have higher levels of caries? A cross-sectional study in Turkish children. Journal of the Indian Society of Pedodontics and Preventive Dentistry. 2007;**25**(2):97-102

[40] Northway WM, Wainright RL, Demirjian A. Effects of premature loss of deciduous molars. The Angle Orthodontist. 1984;**54**(4):295-329

[41] Vellappally S, Gardens SJ, Al Kheraif AA, Krishna M, Babu S, Hashem M, et al. The prevalence of malocclusion and its association with dental caries among 12-18-year-old disabled adolescents. BMC Oral Health. 2014;**14**:123

[42] Stahl F, Grabowski R. Malocclusion and caries prevalence: Is there a connection in the primary and mixed dentitions? Clinical Oral Investigations. 2004;**8**(2):86-90

[43] Onyeaso CO. Comparison of malocclusions and orthodontic treatment needs of handicapped and normal children in Ibadan using the dental aesthetic index (DAI). The Nigerian Postgraduate Medical Journal. 2004;**11**(1):40-44

[44] Baskaradoss JK, Geevarghese A, Roger C, Thaliath A. Prevalence of malocclusion and its relationship with caries among school children aged 11-15 years in southern India. The Korean Journal of Orthodontics. 2013;**43**(1):35-41

[45] Dinesh RB, Arnitha HM, Munshi AK. Malocclusion and orthodontic treatment need of handicapped individuals in South Canara, India. International Dental Journal. 2003;**53**(1):13-18

[46] Hennequin M, Faulks D, Veyrune JL, Bourdiol P. Significance of oral health in persons with down syndrome: A literature review. Developmental Medicine and Child Neurology. 1999;**41**:275-283

[47] Desai SS. Down syndrome: A review of the literature. Oral Surgery, Oral Medicine, Oral Pathology, Oral Radiology, and Endodontics. 1997;**84**:279-285

[48] Oredugba FA. Oral health condition and treatment needs of a group of Nigerian individuals with Down syndrome. Down's Syndrome, Research and Practice. 2007;**12**:72-76

[49] Shore S, Lightfoot T, Ansell P. Oral disease in children with down syndrome: Causes and prevention. Community Practitioner. 2010;**83**:18-21

[50] Zigmond M, Stabholz A, Shapira J, Bachrach G, Chaushu G, Becker A, et al. The outcome of a preventive dental care programme on the prevalence of localized aggressive periodontitis in Down's syndrome individuals. Journal of Intellectual Disability Research. 2006;**50**:492-500

[51] Atsuo A, Jumpei M, Shigehisa A, Morisaki I. Etiologic factors of early-onset in Down syndrome. Japanese Dental Science Review. 2008;**44**: 118-127

[52] Barnett ML, Press KP, Friedman D, Sonnenberg EM. The prevalence of periodontitis and dental caries in a Down's syndrome population. Journal of Periodontology. 1986;**57**:288-293

[53] Stabholz A, Mann J, Sela M, Schurr D, Steinberg D, Shapira J. Caries experience, periodontal treatment needs, salivary pH, and *Streptococcus mutans* counts in a preadolescent Down syndrome population. Special Care in Dentistry. 1991;**11**:203-208

[54] Singh V, Arora R, Bhayya D, Singh D, Sarvaiya B, Mehta D. Comparison of relationship between salivary electrolyte levels and dental caries in children with Down syndrome. Journal of Natural Science, Biology, and Medicine. 2015;**6**(1):144-148

[55] Porovic S, Zukanovic A, Juric H, Dinarevic SM. Oral health of Down syndrome children in Bosnia and Herzegovina. Materia Socio-Medica. 2016;**28**(5):370-372

[56] Shyama M, Al-Mutawa SA, Honkala S. Malocclusions and traumatic injuries in disabled schoolchildren and adolescents in Kuwait. Special Care in Dentistry. 2001;**2**(3):104-108

[57] Oreland A, Heijbel J, Jagell S. Malocclusions in physically and/or mentally handicapped children. Swedish Dental Journal. 1987;**11**(3):103-119

[58] Ondarza A, Jara L, Bertonati MI, Blanco R. Tooth malalignments in Chilean children with Down syndrome. The Cleft Palate-Craniofacial Journal. 1995;**32**(3):188-193

[59] Vittek J, Winik S, Winik A, Sioris C, Tarangelo AM, Chou M. Analysis of orthodontic anomalies in mentally retarded developmentally disabled (MRDD) persons. Special Care in Dentistry. 1994;**14**(5):198-202

[60] Barbaresi WJ, Katustic SK, Voigt RG. Autism: A review of the state of the science for pediatric primary health care clinicians. Archives of Pediatrics & Adolescent Medicine. 2006;**160**(11):1167-1175

[61] Muhle R, Trentacoste SV, Rapin I. The genetics of autism. Pediatrics. 2004;**113**:472-486

[62] Fombonne E. Epidemiology of pervasive developmental disorders. Pediatric Research. 2009;**65**:591-598

[63] Luppanapomplarp S, Leelataweewud P, Putongkam P, Ketanont S. Periodontal status and orthodontic treatment need of autistic children. World Journal of Orthodontics. 2010;**11**(3):256-261

[64] Marshall RI, Bartold PM. A clinical review of drug-induced gingival overgrowths. Australian Dental Journal. 1999;**44**:219-232

[65] Newacheck PW, Hughes DC, Hung YY, Wong S, Stoddard JJ. The unmet health needs of America's children. Pediatrics. 2000;**105**(2): 989-997

[66] Lu YY, Wei IH, Huang CC. Dental health—A challenging problem for a patient with autism spectrum

disorder. General Hospital Psychiatry. 2013;**35**:214-216

[67] Fahlvik PC, Herrstrom P. Dental care of autistic children within the nonspecialized public dental service. Swedish Dental Journal. 2001;**25**:113-118

[68] Desai M, Messer LB, Calache H. A study of the dental treatment needs of children with disabilities in Melbourne, Australia. Australian Dental Journal. 2001;**46**:41-50

[69] Kuter B, Guler N. Caries experience, oral disorders, oral hygiene practices and socio-demographic characteristics of autistic children. European Journal of Paediatric Dentistry. 2019;**20**(3):219-241

[70] Orellana LM, Silvestre FJ, Sanchis SM, Mihi VM, Bautista D. Oral manifestations in a group of adults with autism spectrum disorder. Medicina Oral, Patologia Oral, Cirugia Bucal. 2012;**1**:415-419

[71] Rapin I, Tuchman RF. Autism: Definition, neurobiology, screening, diagnosis. Pediatric Clinics of North America. 2008;**55**:1129-1146

[72] Marshall J, Sheller B, Mancl L. Caries—Risk assessment and caries status of children with autism. Pediatric Dentistry. 2010;**32**(1):69-75

[73] Onol S, Kırzıoğlu Z. Evaluation of oral health status and influential factors in children with autisim. Nigerian Journal of Clinical Practice. 2018;**10**:429-435

[74] Jaber MA, Sayyab M, Abu Fanas SH. Oral health status and dental needs of autistic children and young adults. Journal of Investigative and Clinical Dentistry. 2011;**2**:57-62

[75] Jan MM. Cerebral palsy: Comprehensive review and update. Annals of Saudi Medicine. 2006;**26**:123-132

[76] Gokkaya NK, Caliskan A, Karakus D, Ucan H. Relation between objectively measured growth determinants and ambulation in children with cerebral palsy. Turkish Journal of Medical Sciences. 2009;**39**:85-90

[77] Ortega AO, Guimarães AS, Ciamponi AL, Marie SK. Frequency of parafunctional oral habits in patients with cerebral palsy. Journal of Oral Rehabilitation. 2007;**34**:323-328

[78] Jones MW, Morgan E, Shelton JE. Primary care of the child with cerebral palsy: A review of system (Part II). Journal of Pediatric Health Care. 2007;**21**:226-237

[79] Siegel L, Klingbeil M. Control of drooling with transdermal scopolamine in a child with cerebral palsy. Developmental Medicine and Child Neurology. 1991;**33**:1013-1014

[80] Polat Z, Akgun OM, Turan I, Polat GG, Altun C. Evaluation of the relationship between dental erosion and scintigraphically detected gastroesophageal reflux in patients with cerebral palsy. Turkish Journal of Medical Sciences. 2013;**43**:283-288

[81] Vakil N, van Zanten SV, Kahrilas P, Dent J, Jones R, Global Consensus Group. The Montreal definition and classification of gastroesophageal reflux disease: A global evidence-based consensus. The American Journal of Gastroenterology. 2006;**101**:1900-1920. quiz 1943

[82] Su JM, Tsamtsouris A, Laskou M. Gastroesophageal reflux in children with cerebral palsy and its relationship to erosion of primary and permanent teeth. Journal of the Massachusetts Dental Society. 2003;**52**:20-24

[83] Gonçalves GK, Carmagnani FG, Corrêa MS, Duarte DA, Santos MT. Dental erosion in cerebral palsy patients.

Journal of Dentistry for Children (Chicago, Ill.). 2008;**75**:117-120

[84] Subasi F, Mumcu G, Koksal L, Cimilli H, Bitlis D. Factors affecting oral health habits among children with cerebral palsy: Pilot study. Pediatrics International. 2007;**49**:853-857

[85] Akhter R, Hassan NMM, Martin EF, Muhit M, Smithers-Sheedy H, Badawi N, et al. Caries experience and oral health-related quality of life (OHRQoL) of children and adolescents with cerebral palsy in a low-resource setting. BMC Oral Health. 2019;**19**(1):15

[86] Meningaud JP, Pitak-Arnnop P, Chikhani L, Bertrand JC. Drooling of saliva: A review of the etiology and management options. Oral Surgery, Oral Medicine, Oral Pathology, Oral Radiology, and Endodontics. 2006;**101**:48-57

[87] Holan G, Peretz B, Efrat J, Shapira Y. Traumatic injuries to the teeth in young individuals with cerebral palsy. Dental Traumatology. 2005;**21**:65-69

[88] Lindqvist B, Heijbel J. Bruxism in children with brain damage. Acta Odontologica Scandinavica. 1974;**32**:313-319

[89] Lin X, Wu W, Zhang C, Lo EC, Chu CH, Dissanayaka WL. Prevalence and distribution of developmental enamel defects in children with cerebral palsy in Beijing, China. International Journal of Paediatric Dentistry. 2011;**21**:23-28

[90] Miamoto CB, Pereira LJ, Paiva SM, Pordeus IA, Ramos-Jorge ML, Marques LS. Prevalence and risk indicators of temporomandibular disorder signs and symptoms in a pediatric population with spastic cerebral palsy. The Journal of Clinical Pediatric Dentistry. 2011;**35**(3):259-263